THE COMPLETE BOOK OF KETO

A COMPREHENSIVE GUIDE TO COOKING DELICIOUS AND SATISFYING KETO MEALS

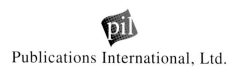

Publications International, Ltd.

Pictured on the front cover *(top to bottom):* Colorful Coleslaw *(page 66)* and Salmon Steaks and Asparagus with Cilantro Pesto *(page 146)*.

Pictured on the back cover *(top to bottom):* Sheet Pan Chicken and Sausage Supper *(page 113)* and Greek Salad *(page 70)*.

Photographs on front cover (bottom) and pages 69, 75 and 147 copyright © Shutterstock.com.

Contributing Writer: Jacqueline B. Marcus, MS, RDN, LDN, CNS, FADA, FAND

ISBN: 978-1-64558-206-9

Manufactured in China.

8 7 6 5 4 3 2 1

Microwave Cooking: Microwave ovens vary in wattage. Use the cooking times as guidelines and check for doneness before adding more time.

Let's get social!

⊙ @Publications_International

⬛ @PublicationsInternational

www.pilcookbooks.com

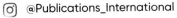

TABLE OF
CONTENTS

INTRODUCTION

DIETARY FATS AND OILS, WEIGHT AND HEALTH

Want to hear some good news about dietary fats and oils—especially how they relate to weight and health?

Consuming dietary fats and oils is not as bad as you might think—nor will consuming dietary fats and oils necessarily make you fat. The right amounts and types of dietary fats and oils may actually be satisfying and contribute to weight loss and weight maintenance. Dietary fats and oils are essential to your overall diet. Understanding what dietary fats and oils are and how they fit into an overall diet will help you with food selection, preparation and meal and menu planning.

The keto diet is based on ketones, organic compounds that are produced when dietary carbohydrates are limited. Ketosis is a normal metabolic process whereby the body burns stored fats instead of glucose from carbohydrates for energy. A diet based on ketosis, with its abundance of dietary fats and oils may actually help your dieting efforts. Understanding more about ketones and their place in a ketogenic diet may assist your food choices and dietary efforts.

In addition to their role in weight loss and weight management, different types of dietary fats and oils and ketones are important for brain function, some disease protection and management, and overall health if used advantageously and correctly.

Dietary fats and oils are naturally found in foods and beverages such as dairy products, eggs, nuts, meats and seeds. Manufactured dietary fats and oils are found in some beverages, processed foods like margarine, cheeses and meats. Ketones are produced by the human body—you'll soon discover how.

There are differing viewpoints on the benefits of different types of dietary fats and oils and about ketones, the ideal amounts to consume and how ketones may sensibly be used for weight loss.

The purpose of this book is to help educate you about the types of dietary and blood fats and their contribution to health, and their relation to ketones and the ketogenic diet. It provides you with recipes that focus on healthy fats, proteins and non-starchy vegetables and de-emphasizes carbohydrates—particularly those that are refined or processed.

Your healthcare provider may help you determine if these approaches to eating and dieting are appropriate for you, so ask your doctor before you begin this or any other diet program.

Choose the Right Fats

Fats are essential for proper body functioning and contribute satisfaction to diets, plus fats add flavor to foods and beverages. Still, fats provide more than twice the number of calories as carbohydrates or proteins (9 calories per gram compared to 4 calories per gram respectively). On a ketogenic diet, there is a different approach to fats than other diets that may restrict fats. The key is to understand the importance of fats in ketogenic diets and how to use them to your advantage.

> **The key is to understand the importance of fats in ketogenic diets AND how to use them to your advantage.**

Types of Fats

Saturated fats are primarily found in foods from animal sources, such as meat, poultry and full-fat dairy products, while trans fats are mostly created when oils are partially hydrogenated to improve their cooking applications and to give them a longer shelf life. Saturated and trans fats may place a person at greater risk for heart disease. On the other hand, unsaturated fats that include monounsaturated and polyunsaturated fatty acids, found in plant-based foods such as avocados, nuts and seeds and olives and olive oil, and in fatty fish such as salmon, sardines and tuna tend to lower the risk of heart issues.

The American Heart Association (AHA) Diet and Lifestyle Recommendations suggest that a person limit saturated and trans fats and replace them with monounsaturated and polyunsaturated fats. If blood cholesterol needs to be lowered, then the recommendation is to reduce saturated fat to no more than 5 to 6 percent of total calories. For someone consuming 2,000 calories a day, this is about 13 grams of saturated fat, or about 117 calories. This is the equivalent of about 1 ounce of Cheddar cheese (9.4% total fat with 6 grams of saturated fat) and about 3 ounces of regular ground beef (25% total fat with 6.1 grams of saturated fat).

Try to eliminate trans fats (fats that have been processed into saturated fats) completely, or limit them to less than 1 percent of total daily calories. On a 2,000-calorie diet, this means that fewer than 20 calories (about 2 grams) should be derived from trans fats.

THE KETOGENIC DIET AND DIETING

The ketogenic diet is hardly new. The idea that fasting could be used as a therapy to treat disease was one that ancient Greek and Indian physicians embraced. "On the Sacred Disease," an early treatise in the Hippocratic Corpus, proposed how dietary modifications could be useful in epileptic management. Hippocrates, a Greek physician called the Father of Modern Medicine, wrote in "Epidemics" how abstinence from food and drink cured epilepsy.

In the 20th century, the first ketogenic diet became popularized in the 1920's and 30's as a regimen for treating epilepsy and an alternative to non-mainstream fasting. It was also promoted as a means of restoring health. In 1921, the ketogenic diet was officially established when an endocrinologist noted that three water-soluble compounds were produced by the liver as a result of following a diet that was rich in fat and low in carbohydrates. The term "water diet" had been used prior to this time to describe a diet that was free of starch and sugar. This is because when carbohydrates are broken down by the body carbon dioxide and water are by-products. When newer, anticonvulsant therapies were established, the ketogenic diet was temporarily abandoned.

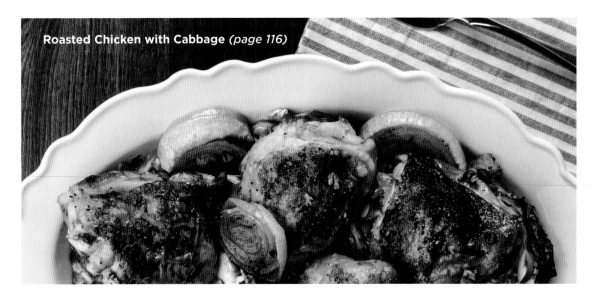

Roasted Chicken with Cabbage *(page 116)*

TABLE 1

KETOGENIC DIET BASICS

Generally, the percentages of macronutrients on a ketogenic diet are as follows:

- Fat 60 to 75 percent of total daily calories
- Protein 15 to 30 percent of total daily calories
- Carbohydrates 5 to 10 percent of total daily calories

Both fat and protein have high priority on a ketogenic diet, with non-starchy carbohydrates completing the remaining calories. While calories are not as important on the ketogenic diet as they are for other diets, a closer examination of the contributions of these macronutrients helps to put the amounts into perspective.

If total daily calories were about 2,000, then the percentages of macronutrients on a ketogenic diet would resemble the following amounts:

- Fat 60 to 75 percent of total daily calories or about 1,200 to 1,500 calories
- Protein 15 to 30 percent of total daily calories or about 300 to 600 calories
- Carbohydrates 5 to 10 percent of total daily calories or about 100 to 200 calories

In selecting foods and beverages, think protein and fat first, then non-starchy carbohydrates to complete. Until you truly have a handle on what constitutes low carbohydrates, find a carbohydrate counter to help to keep you in line. The ketogenic diet meal suggestions in **Table 5 – SAMPLE KETOGENIC DIET MEALS: BREAKFAST, LUNCH, DINNER AND SNACKS** on page 15 may help your food and beverage selections.

In the 1960's the ketogenic diet was revisited when it was noted that more ketones are produced by medium chain triglycerides (MCTs) per unit of energy than by normal dietary fats (mostly long-chain triglycerides) because MCTs are quickly transported to the liver to be metabolized. In research diets where about 60 percent of the calories came from MCT oil, more protein and up to about three times as many carbohydrates could be consumed in comparison to "classic" ketogenic diets. This is why MCT oil is included in some ketogenic diets today.

In the 1950's and 1960's many versions of the ketogenic diet were popularized as high-protein, low-carbohydrate and a quick method of weight loss. Also at this time, the risk factors of excess fat and protein in the diet were criticized for being detrimental to health. Outside of the medical community, the ketogenic diet was not widely recognized for its therapeutic benefits so response to it was sensational in scope.

TABLE 2

ADVANTAGES AND DRAWBACKS OF KETOGENIC DIETS

ADVANTAGES

- No calorie counting or focus on portion sizes
- Initial weight loss
- After initial transition, hunger subsides
- Improved energy
- Improved blood pressure
- Improved blood fats: high-density lipoproteins, cholesterol, low-density lipoproteins, triglycerides
- Reduced blood sugar, C-reactive protein (marker of inflammation), insulin, waist circumference
- Significant short-term weight loss possible

DRAWBACKS

- Hard to sustain
- Limited food choices
- May lead to taste fatigue
- Socialization difficult
- Digestive issues (such as constipation, fatty stool, nausea)
- Nutrient deficiencies (such as calcium, vitamins A, C and D, B-vitamins, fiber, magnesium, selenium)
- Fiber, vitamin and mineral supplements suggested
- Increased urination (bladder, kidney contraindications)
- Diabetes issues
- Rapid, sizeable short-term weight loss concerning; long-term weight maintenance questionable

Then in the 1980's the Glycemic Index (GI) of foods and beverages was revealed that accounted for the differences in the speed of digestion of different types of carbohydrates. This explanation became the springboard for a number of ketogenic diets that were revised from years earlier. By the late 1990's the low-carb craze became one of the most popular types of dieting. Since this time, the original ketogenic diet underwent many refinements and hybrid diets developed.

Variations of the ketogenic diet continued to surface throughout the 20th century since the premise of the ketogenic diet—higher fat and protein and low carbohydrate—was used to treat diabetes and induce weight loss among other applications.

Table 1 summarizes the ketogenic diet basics. Many clinical studies examined their effectiveness and safety and their advantages and drawbacks were identified. These are condensed in Table 2.

> One of the most important roles of fat in the body is as an energy source, especially when carbohydrates are not available from the diet or are lacking in the body.

FAT IN HEALTH AND DISEASE

Fats are essential to the diet and health for many purposes. Fats function as the body's thermostat. The layer of fat just beneath the skin helps to keep the body warm or causes it to perspire to cool the body.

Fat contributes to bile acids, cell membranes and steroid hormones (such as estrogen and testosterone), cushions the body from shock and helps to regulate fluid balance. Too many or too few fats in the diet may influence each of these important body functions.

One of the most important roles of fat in the body is as an energy source, especially when carbohydrates are not available from the diet or are lacking in the body. When people did manual work all day and expended the calories that they consumed, they made good use of carbohydrates and fats in their diet and within their energy stores. Today's laborsaving devices and sedentary lifestyles create less need for excess carbohydrate calories—particularly if they are refined. Even a plant-based diet may be unnecessarily high in refined carbohydrate calories.

Over the years, as humans moved from a plant-based diet toward an animal-based diet, the composition of fatty acids in the American diet switched from monounsaturated and polyunsaturated fats to more saturated fats, which are associated more with cardiovascular disease. A diet that is only filled with saturated fats may not be healthy. Incorporating avocado, fish, nuts, oils and seeds and other foods that contain monounsaturated and polyunsaturated fats into your diet may help to support a healthier proportion of fats in the body for weight maintenance and good health.

Besides cardiovascular disease, excess saturated and trans fats in the human diet are associated with certain cancers, cerebral vascular disease, diabetes, obesity and metabolic syndrome (a collection of conditions that may include abnormal

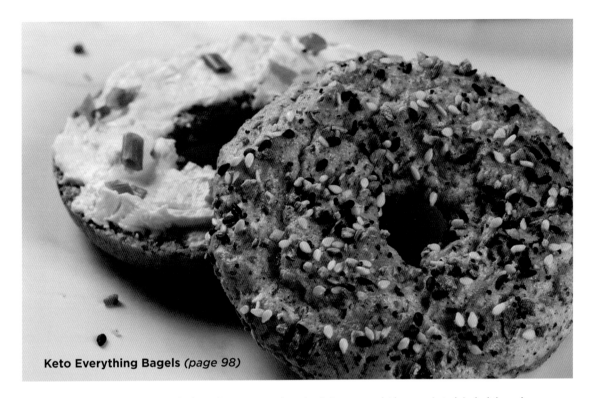

Keto Everything Bagels *(page 98)*

cholesterol or triglyceride levels, excess body fat around the waist, high blood sugar and increased blood pressure that may increase a person's risk of diabetes, heart disease and/or stroke).

The Cholesterol Controversy

Atherosclerosis, or hardening of the arteries, is not a modern disease. Rather, the association between blood cholesterol and cardiovascular disease was recognized as far back as the 1850's.

One hundred years later in the 1950's, cholesterol and saturated fats in the diet were implicated as major risk factors for cardiovascular disease. Then in the 1980's, major US health institutions established that the process of lowering blood cholesterol (specifically LDL-cholesterol) reduces the risk of heart attacks that are caused by coronary heart disease.

Some scientists questioned this conclusion that marked the unofficial start of what's been called the "cholesterol controversy." Studies of cholesterol-lowering drugs known as statins supported the idea that reducing blood cholesterol means less mortality from heart disease. Subsequent statin studies have questioned this association. Other factors aside from dietary cholesterol have since been identified that may lead to elevated blood cholesterol, such as trans fats.

The liver manufactures cholesterol, so reducing cholesterol in the diet should help to reduce blood cholesterol, coronary heart disease and the risk of heart attack. But in some individuals, the liver produces more cholesterol than the body requires and cardiovascular disease may still develop. Accordingly, dietary cholesterol does not necessarily predict cardiovascular disease or a heart attack.

> What you'll likely end up with is a satisfying eating plan with ample protein, healthy fats **AND** minimal carbohydrates that may help you to feel full **AND** lose weight in the process.

While dietary cholesterol may be a measure for greater cardiovascular risks, cardiovascular disease and heart attacks are also dependent upon such lifestyle and genetic factors as age, diet, exercise, gender, genetics, medication and stress. Reducing hydrogenated fats, saturated fats and trans fats; incorporating mono- and polyunsaturated fats and losing weight to help better manage blood fats are other sensible measures to take.

Longer-term weight management is also a preventative measure in cardiovascular disease. Reducing cholesterol and saturated fat in the diet while integrating foods and beverages with mono- and polyunsaturated fats and oils, dietary fiber, antioxidants and other phytonutrients may lead to a decrease in overall calorie consumption and weight loss and an improvement in overall health.

SO WHAT (AND HOW) SHOULD I EAT?

If you want to lose body fat, then the general consensus is that you need to take in fewer calories than you burn for energy. For example, if you're an average woman over 40, decreasing your caloric intake may be a reasonable starting point. If you are of shorter stature and/or very inactive, or you haven't dropped any pounds after a few weeks, you may consider lowering your daily intake of calories by 100-calorie increments until you start seeing weight loss. But don't go much below 1,000 calories

TABLE 3

ACCEPTABLE FOODS, BEVERAGES AND INGREDIENTS FOR KETOGENIC DIETS

BEVERAGES

- Broth
- Hard liquor
- Nut milks
- Unsweetened coffee, tea
- Water

EGGS

- Egg whites
- Powdered eggs
- Whole eggs

FATS AND OILS

- Butter
- Cocoa butter
- Coconut butter, cream and oil
- Ghee
- Lard
- Oils: avocado oil, macadamia nut oil, MCT oil, olive oil and cold-pressed vegetable oils (flax, safflower, soybean)
- Mayonnaise

FISH AND SEAFOOD

- Anchovies
- Fish (catfish, cod, flounder, halibut, mackerel, mahi-mahi, salmon, snapper, trout, tuna)
- Shellfish (clams, crab, lobster, mussels, oysters, scallops, squid)

FRUITS AND VEGETABLES

- Avocados
- Cruciferous vegetables (broccoli, brussels sprouts, cabbage, cauliflower, kohlrabi)
- Fermented vegetables (kimchi, sauerkraut)
- Leafy greens (bok choy, chard, endive, lettuce, kale, radicchio, spinach, watercress)
- Lemon and lime juice and peel
- Mushrooms
- Non-starchy vegetables (asparagus, bamboo shoots, celery, cucumber)
- Seaweed and kelp
- Squash (spaghetti squash, yellow squash, zucchini)
- Tomatoes (used in moderation in some keto diets)

DAIRY PRODUCTS

- Crème fraîche
- Greek yogurt
- Hard cheese (aged Cheddar, feta, Parmesan, Swiss)
- Heavy cream
- Soft cheese (Brie, blue, Colby, Monterey Jack, mozzarella)
- Sour cream
- Spreadable cheese (cream cheese, cottage cheese and mascarpone)

MEATS AND POULTRY

- Beef (ground beef, roasts, steak, stew meat)
- Goat (leg, loin, rack, saddle, shoulder)
- Lamb (leg, loin, rack, ribs, shank, shoulder)
- Organ meats (heart, kidneys, liver, tongue)
- Poultry with skin (such as chicken, duck, pheasant, quail, turkey)
- Pork (bacon and sausage without fillers, ground pork, ham, pork chops, pork loin, tenderloin)
- Tofu used in moderation in some keto diets)
- Veal (double, flank, leg, rib, shoulder, sirloin)

NON-DAIRY BEVERAGES

- Almond milk
- Cashew milk
- Coconut milk
- Soymilk (used in moderation in some keto diets)

NUTS AND SEEDS

- Nut butters (almond, macadamia)
- Seeds (chia, flax, poppy, sesame, sunflower)
- Whole nuts (almonds, Brazil nuts, macadamia, pecans, hazelnuts, pine nuts, walnuts)

PANTRY ITEMS

- Herbs (dried or fresh such as basil, cilantro, oregano, parsley, rosemary and thyme)
- Horseradish
- Hot sauce
- Mustard
- Pepper
- Pesto sauce
- Pickles
- Salad dressings (without sweeteners)
- Salt
- Spices (such as ground red pepper, chili powder, cinnamon and cumin)
- Unsweetened gelatin
- Vinegar
- Whey protein (unsweetened)
- Worcestershire sauce

TABLE 4

UNACCEPTABLE FOODS, BEVERAGES AND INGREDIENTS FOR KETOGENIC DIETS

- Alcohol other than hard liquor (beer, sugary alcoholic beverages, wine)
- Beans
- Breads and breadstuffs
- Cakes and pastries
- Candy
- Cereals
- Cookies
- Crackers
- Flours
- Fruit, all (fresh, dried)

- Grains (amaranth, barley, buckwheat, bulgur, corn, millet, oats, rice, rye, sorghum, sprouted grains, wheat)
- Legumes (lentils, peas)
- Margarines with trans fats
- Milk (full-fat milk is acceptable in some ketogenic diets)
- Oats and muesli
- Potatoes, all kinds (white, yellow, sweet)
- Quinoa

- Pasta
- Pizza
- Processed and refined snack foods
- Rice
- Root vegetables
- Soda
- Sports drinks
- Sugar and honey
- Syrup
- Wheat gluten
- Yams

without your health care provider's supervision. (And be sure to check with your health care provider before making any major changes to your diet or activity level, especially if you have any serious health problems.)

Another approach to weight loss is the ketogenic diet that does not focus on calories. Instead, the ketogenic diet focuses on the composition of calories from fats, proteins and carbohydrates.

Fats are satisfying because they take longer for the body to digest, and some are converted into ketones for energy. You don't want to skimp on proteins because protein helps maintain and build calorie-burning muscle and also keeps you satiated between meals. Choose protein sources that supply monounsaturated fats and other heart-healthy unsaturated fats; good options include fish, seafood, nuts and seeds. (Fatty fish, such as herring, mackerel, salmon and tuna contain polyunsaturated fats—especially disease-fighting omega-3 fatty acids). You'll need to replace highly processed and refined foods that are full of saturated and trans fats, sugar and refined carbohydrates with minimally processed fiber- and nutrient-rich foods that include non-starchy vegetables.

What you'll likely end up with is a satisfying eating plan with ample protein, healthy fats and minimal carbohydrates that may help you to feel full and lose weight in the process. It's also a plan that may help you to maintain weight loss over time in a modified manner.

If you've ever tried to lose weight before, you know how quickly between-meal hunger may sabotage your best efforts. When your stomach starts rumbling hours before your next meal, it's tempting to grab whatever is available. Often, that "whatever" is some unhealthy packaged snack food or beverage that is loaded with empty calories, sodium, sugars and/or unhealthy fats. Or, if you manage to ignore this hunger, you may become so ravenous at the next meal that you consume far more calories than your body actually needs.

To prevent hunger from spoiling your weight-loss efforts, eat when you are hungry and stop eating when you are full, whether a meal or snack. Try to consume meals and snacks that include a source of hunger-fighting protein and healthy fat, and count your carbs so as not to exceed the daily limit of 20 to 50 grams of non-starchy carbohydrates.

Drink plenty of water throughout the day (especially if you live in a hot climate or sweat excessively) since ketogenic diets tend to be dehydrating and may lead to fatigue or ill feelings. This may be due to an imbalance of electrolytes; specifically sodium that the kidneys excrete during ketosis. Sometimes lightly salting your food may help to restore sodium. A high-quality vitamin and mineral supplement is also sensible.

NOTES ON KETOGENIC FOODS, BEVERAGES AND INGREDIENTS

In general, the foods, beverages and ingredients that are included in a ketogenic diet incorporate eggs, healthy fats and oils, fish, meats and organ meats and non-starchy vegetables. These "acceptable" foods, beverages and ingredients contain protein and fats and are low in carbohydrates that contribute to the effectiveness of ketogenic diets. They are listed in **Table 3 – ACCEPTABLE FOODS, BEVERAGES AND INGREDIENTS FOR KETOGENIC DIETS.**

In **Table 4 – UNACCEPTABLE FOODS, BEVERAGES AND INGREDIENTS FOR KETOGENIC DIETS** are shown. While there is a wide-range of ketogenic diet approaches, these foods, beverages and ingredients are generally considered to be "unacceptable" on many ketogenic diets. In general, their carbohydrate content exceeds what is considered as optimal for effective ketosis and diet success.

TABLE 5

SAMPLE KETOGENIC DIET MEALS: BREAKFAST, LUNCH, DINNER AND SNACKS

Examples of combinations of protein, low-carb, non-starchy vegetables and fats:

BREAKFAST:

- Almond, coconut, hemp or other nut or seed milks or beverages (unsweetened)
- Bacon, sausage or sliced meats (without carbohydrate fillers)
- Cheese, hard or soft varieties
- Eggs, scrambled or fried + vegetables (asparagus, broccoli, garlic, mushrooms, onions or spinach) + coconut or olive oil + avocado, olives, salsa and/or sour cream
- Greek yogurt with nut butter, chia or flax seeds, herbs and spices (cinnamon, ginger or nutmeg)
- Smoked fish (such as lox, sable or whitefish)
- Smoothies made with keto-friendly ingredients (protein powder, almond or coconut butter, avocado, cocoa powder, chia or flax seeds, spices such as cinnamon, smoked paprika or turmeric and unsweetened almond or hemp milk)
- Vegetable slices (cucumber or zucchini or lettuce) topped with cheese

LUNCH AND DINNER:

- Eggs + watercress or spinach + avocado dressing
- Lamb + kale + sesame oil
- Pork + cauliflower + coconut butter
- Poultry + zucchini and yellow squash + extra virgin olive oil
- Salmon + broccoli + mustard sauce
- Sardines + cucumbers and onions + sour cream dressing
- Seafood + leafy green salad + oil and vinegar dressing
- Steak + asparagus + butter sauce
- Tofu + mushrooms and bok choy + ghee
- Tuna + celery + mayonnaise

SNACKS:

- Asparagus with goat cheese dip
- Avocado filled hard-cooked eggs
- Celery + nut or seed butter
- Cheese + olive skewers
- Chia and flaxseed crackers + cream cheese
- Cucumber and cream cheese spread
- Cream cheese and bacon stuffed celery
- Deviled eggs with fresh herbs and chives
- Greek yogurt with chopped cucumbers and garlic
- Guacamole with onions and garlic
- Ham and Cheddar or Swiss cheese roll ups
- Mixed nut-coated cheese balls
- Nut butters (such as almond) blended with ricotta cheese
- Olives stuffed with blue cheese
- Parmesan cheese crisps
- Seeds and seed butters such as tahini
- Sliced jicama with herbed cream cheese

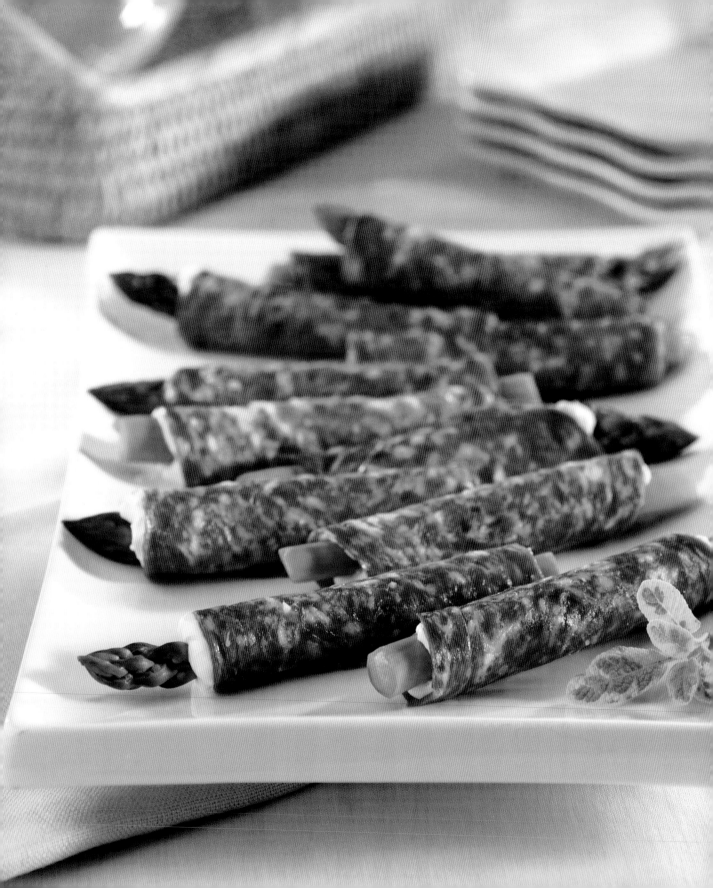

SNACKS
AND SOUPS

ASPARAGUS ROLL-UPS
MAKES ABOUT 24 ROLL-UPS

1 pound asparagus,
   tough ends trimmed
   (about 24 spears)
½ teaspoon salt
4 ounces cream cheese,
   softened
½ pound thinly sliced
   salami

1 Cut asparagus into lengths 1 inch longer than width of salami. Reserve bottoms for another use.

2 Place about ½ inch of water in large skillet; add salt. Bring to a simmer over medium heat. Add asparagus; simmer 4 to 5 minutes or until crisp-tender. Drain and immediately immerse in cold water to stop cooking. Drain and pat dry with paper towel.

3 Spread about 1 teaspoon cream cheese evenly over one side of each salami slice. Roll up 1 asparagus spear in each salami slice.

4 Cover and refrigerate until ready to serve. Let stand at room temperature 10 minutes before serving.

NUTRIENTS PER SERVING (SERVING SIZE: 1 ROLL-UP)

CALORIES 40   **TOTAL FAT** 3g   **CARBS** 1g   **NET CARBS** 1g   **DIETARY FIBER** 0g   **PROTEIN** 2g

MOZZARELLA & PROSCIUTTO BITES

MAKES 16 TO 20 PIECES

16 to 20 small bamboo skewers or toothpicks

1 ball (8 ounces) fresh mozzarella

¼ cup chopped fresh basil

½ teaspoon black pepper

6 to 8 thin prosciutto slices

1 Soak skewers in water 20 minutes to prevent burning. Cut mozzarella into 1- to 1½-inch chunks.* Place on paper towel-lined plate; sprinkle with basil and pepper, turning to coat all sides.

2 Cut prosciutto slices crosswise into thirds. Tightly wrap one prosciutto slice around each piece of mozzarella, covering completely. Insert skewer into each piece; place on cutting board. Freeze 15 minutes to firm.

3 Preheat broiler. Line broiler pan or baking sheet with foil. Place skewers on prepared pan; broil about 3 minutes or until prosciutto begins to crisp, turning once. Serve immediately.

Or substitute one 8-ounce container of small fresh mozzarella balls (ciliengini). One 8-ounce container contains 24 balls.

NUTRIENTS PER SERVING (SERVING SIZE: 1 PIECE)

CALORIES 50 **TOTAL FAT** 4g **CARBS** 0g **NET CARBS** 0g **DIETARY FIBER** 0g **PROTEIN** 4g

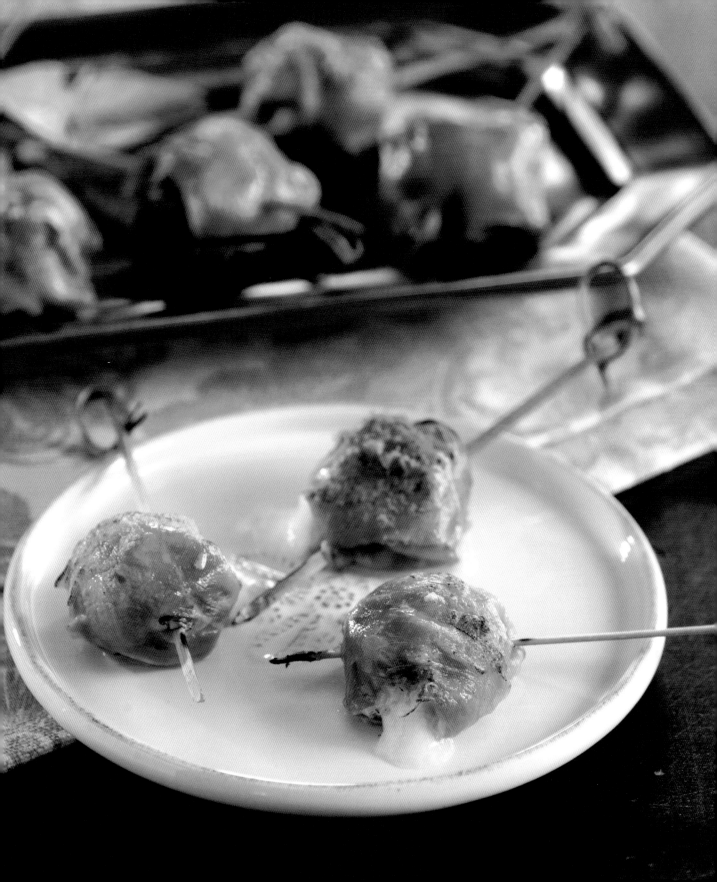

CHILLED CUCUMBER SOUP
MAKES 4 SERVINGS

1 large cucumber, peeled and coarsely chopped
¾ cup sour cream
¼ cup packed fresh dill
½ teaspoon salt
⅛ teaspoon white pepper (optional)
1½ cups vegetable broth

1 Place cucumber in food processor; process until finely chopped. Add sour cream, dill, salt and white pepper, if desired; process until fairly smooth.

2 Transfer mixture to large bowl; stir in broth. Cover and refrigerate at least 2 hours or up to 24 hours before serving.

NUTRIENTS PER SERVING (SERVING SIZE: ¾ CUP SOUP)

CALORIES 67   TOTAL FAT 4g   CARBS 6g   NET CARBS 5g   DIETARY FIBER 1g   PROTEIN 3g

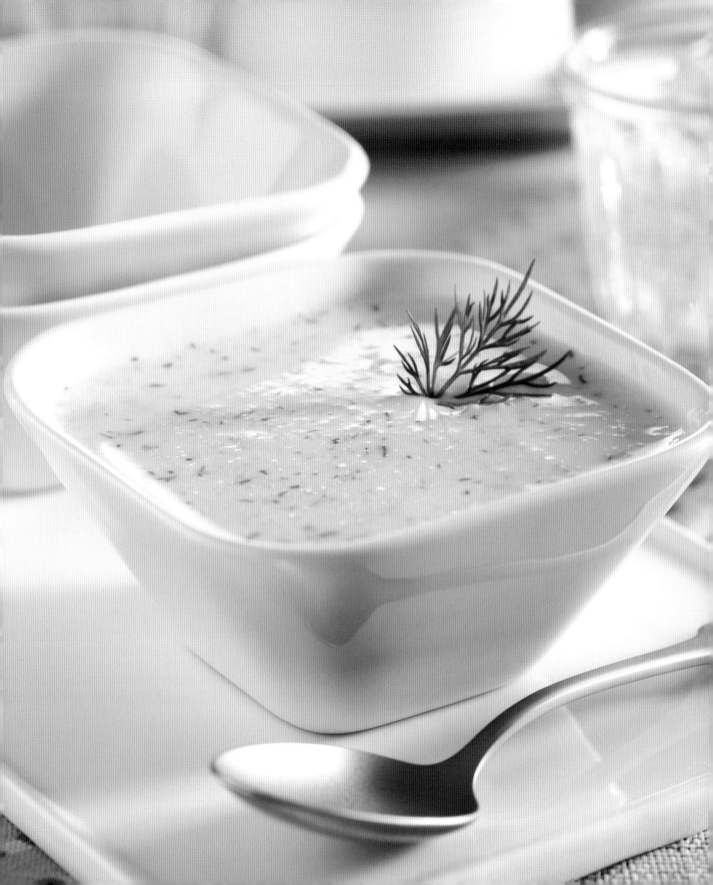

CLASSIC DEVILED EGGS

MAKES 12 DEVILED EGGS

6 eggs

3 tablespoons mayonnaise

½ teaspoon apple cider vinegar

½ teaspoon yellow mustard

⅛ teaspoon salt

Optional toppings: black pepper, paprika, minced chives and/or minced red onion (optional)

1 Bring medium saucepan of water to a boil. Gently add eggs with slotted spoon. Reduce heat to maintain a simmer; cook 12 minutes. Meanwhile, fill medium bowl with cold water and ice cubes. Drain eggs and place in ice water; cool 10 minutes.

2 Carefully peel eggs. Cut eggs in half; place yolks in small bowl. Add mayonnaise, vinegar, mustard and salt; mash until well blended. Spoon mixture into egg whites; garnish with desired toppings.

NUTRIENTS PER SERVING (SERVING SIZE: 1 DEVILED EGG)

CALORIES 30 **TOTAL FAT** 3g **CARBS** 0g **NET CARBS** 0g **DIETARY FIBER** 0g **PROTEIN** 2g

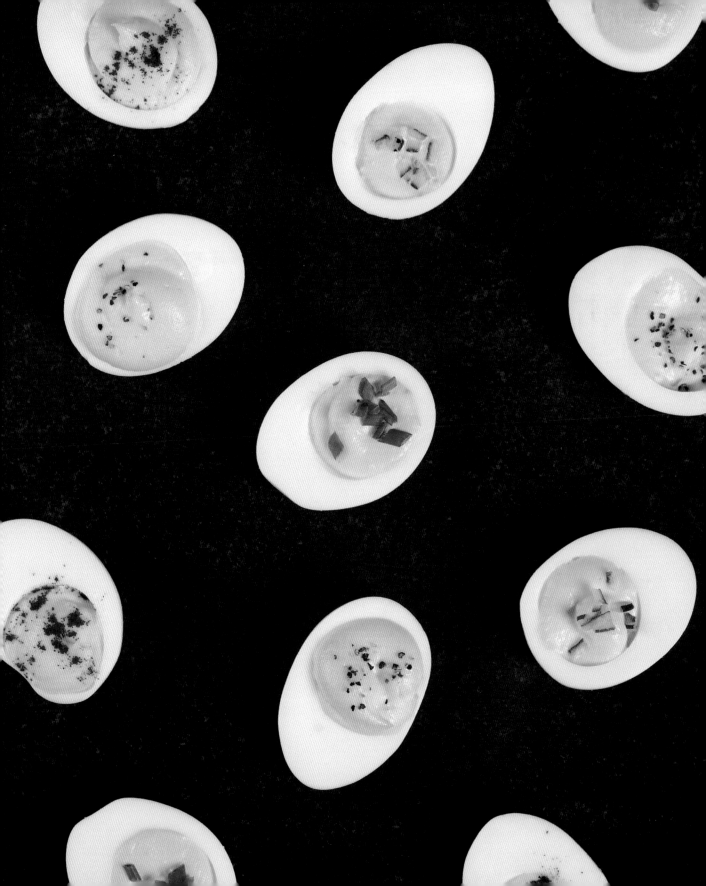

JALAPEÑO POPPERS

MAKES 20 TO 24 POPPERS

10 to 12 fresh jalapeño peppers*

1 package (8 ounces) cream cheese, softened

1½ cups (6 ounces) shredded Cheddar cheese, divided

2 green onions, finely chopped

½ teaspoon onion powder

¼ teaspoon salt

⅛ teaspoon garlic powder

6 slices bacon, crisp-cooked and finely chopped

2 tablespoons almond flour (optional)

2 tablespoons grated Parmesan or Romano cheese

For large jalapeño peppers, use 10. For small peppers, use 12.

1 Preheat oven to 375°F. Line baking sheet with parchment paper or foil.

2 Cut each jalapeño in half lengthwise; remove ribs and seeds.

3 Combine cream cheese, 1 cup Cheddar cheese, green onions, onion powder, salt and garlic powder in medium bowl. Stir in bacon. Fill each jalapeño half with about 1 tablespoon cheese mixture. Place on prepared baking sheet. Sprinkle with remaining ½ cup Cheddar cheese, almond flour, if desired, and Parmesan cheese.

4 Bake 10 to 12 minutes or until cheese is melted but jalapeños are still firm.

NUTRIENTS PER SERVING (SERVING SIZE: 1 POPPER)

CALORIES 110 **TOTAL FAT** 10g **CARBS** 2g **NET CARBS** 2g **DIETARY FIBER** 0g **PROTEIN** 4g

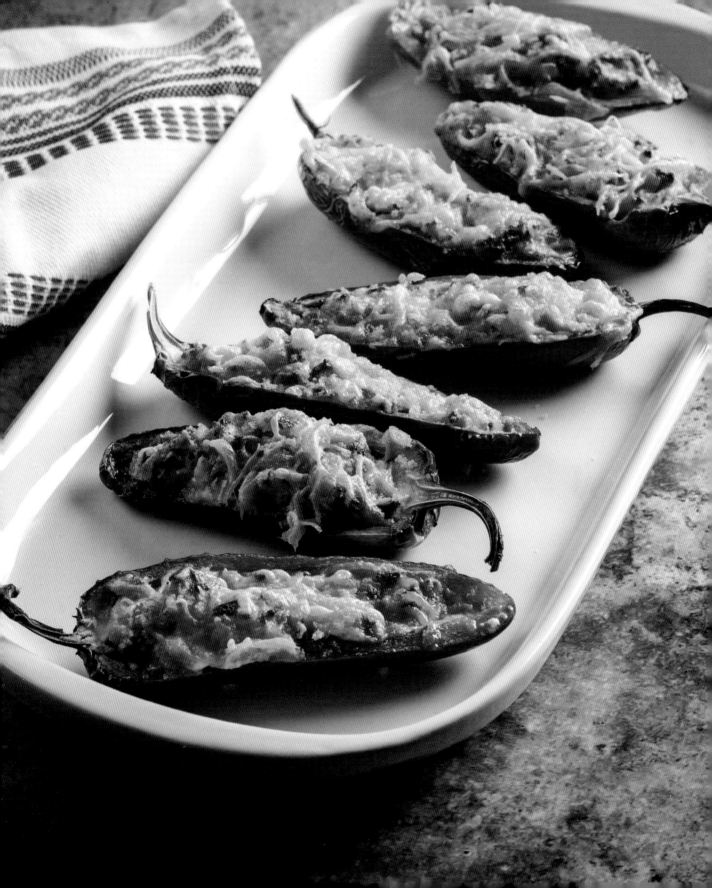

ROMAN SPINACH SOUP

MAKES 8 SERVINGS

6 cups chicken broth

1 cup liquid egg
    substitute

¼ cup minced fresh basil

3 tablespoons grated
    Parmesan cheese

2 tablespoons fresh
    lemon juice

1 tablespoon minced
    fresh parsley

¼ teaspoon white pepper

⅛ teaspoon ground
    nutmeg

8 cups packed fresh
    spinach, chopped

1 Bring broth to a boil in 4-quart saucepan over medium
heat.

2 Whisk egg substitute, basil, Parmesan, lemon juice,
parsley, white pepper and nutmeg in small bowl.

3 Stir spinach into broth; simmer 1 minute. Slowly pour
egg mixture into broth mixture, whisking constantly so
egg threads form. Simmer 2 to 3 minutes or until egg is
cooked (soup may look curdled). Serve immediately.

NUTRIENTS PER SERVING (SERVING SIZE: ¾ CUP SOUP)

CALORIES 46   **TOTAL FAT** 1g   **CARBS** 4g   **NET CARBS** 3g   **DIETARY FIBER** 1g   **PROTEIN** 6g

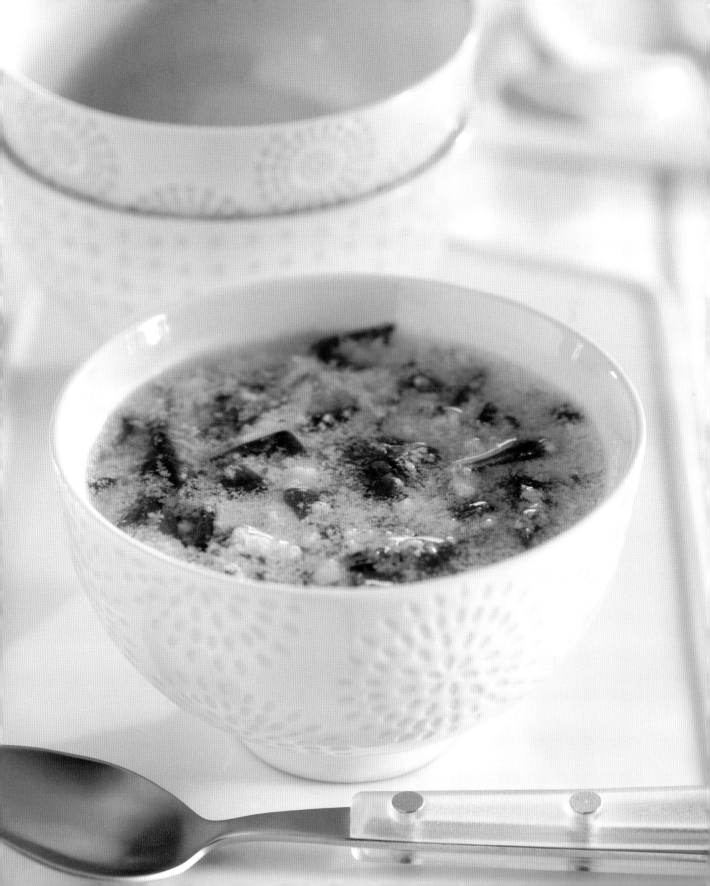

QUICK AND EASY STUFFED MUSHROOMS
MAKES 8 SERVINGS

16 large mushrooms
½ cup sliced celery
½ cup sliced onion
1 clove garlic
½ cup almond flour
1 teaspoon
    Worcestershire
    sauce
½ teaspoon dried
    marjoram
⅛ teaspoon ground red
    pepper
    Dash paprika

1 Preheat oven to 350°F. Remove stems from mushrooms; reserve caps. Place mushroom stems, celery, onion and garlic in food processor; pulse until vegetables are finely chopped.

2 Spray large skillet with nonstick cooking spray; heat over medium heat. Add vegetable mixture; cook and stir 5 minutes or until onion is tender. Transfer to bowl. Stir in almond flour, Worcestershire sauce, marjoram and red pepper.

3 Fill mushroom caps evenly with mixture, pressing down firmly. Place about ½ inch apart in shallow baking pan. Spray tops with nonstick cooking spray. Sprinkle with paprika.

4 Bake 15 minutes or until heated through.

NOTE

Mushrooms can be stuffed up to 1 day ahead. Cover and refrigerate filled mushroom caps until ready to serve. Bake in preheated 300°F oven 20 minutes or until heated through.

NUTRIENTS PER SERVING (SERVING SIZE: 2 STUFFED MUSHROOM CAPS)

CALORIES 50   **TOTAL FAT** 4g   **CARBS** 4g   **NET CARBS** 3g   **DIETARY FIBER** 1g   **PROTEIN** 2g

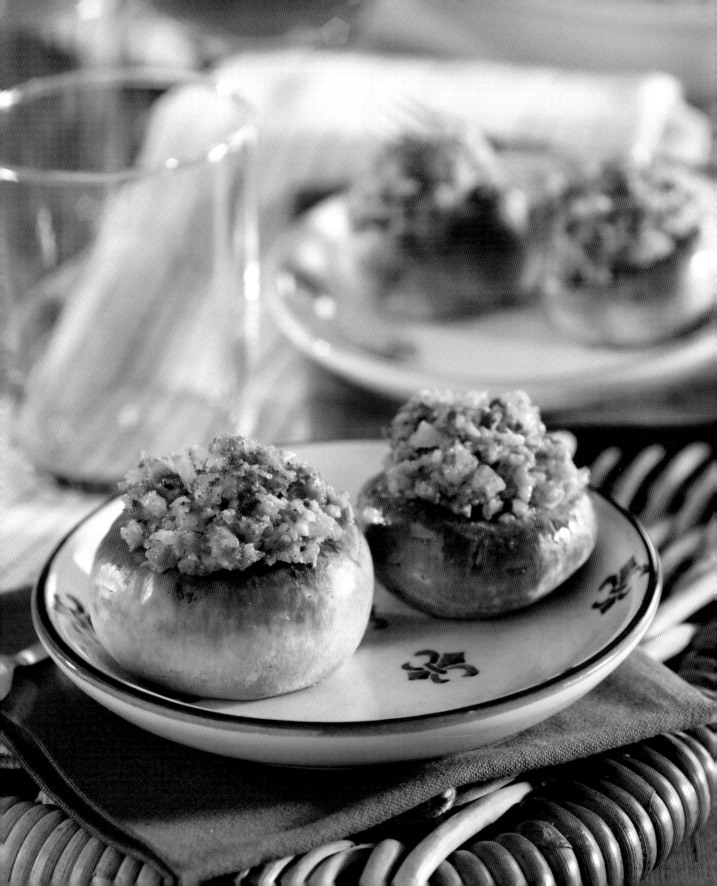

GARLIC "BREAD" STICKS

MAKES 14 STICKS

- 1 medium head cauliflower, finely chopped
- 1 cup (4 ounces) shredded mozzarella cheese
- 1 cup shredded Parmesan cheese, divided
- ¾ cup almond flour
- 2 cloves garlic, minced
- ½ teaspoon Italian seasoning
- 1 teaspoon salt
- 1 egg

  Tomato sauce or pizza sauce for dipping (optional)

1 Preheat oven to 425°F. Grease sheet pan with 1 tablespoon olive oil or line with parchment paper.

2 Squeeze excess moisture from cauliflower between layers of paper towels. Combine cauliflower, mozzarella, ½ cup Parmesan, almond flour, garlic, Italian seasoning, salt and egg in large bowl; mix well. Pat into 12×10-inch rectangle on prepared sheet pan.

3 Bake 30 minutes or until well browned and edges are crispy. Sprinkle with remaining ½ cup Parmesan. Bake 10 minutes or until cheese is melted. Cool slightly. Cut into sticks to serve. Serve with tomato sauce for dipping, if desired.

NUTRIENTS PER SERVING (SERVING SIZE: 1 STICK)

CALORIES 110 **TOTAL FAT** 8g **CARBS** 4g **NET CARBS** 3g **DIETARY FIBER** 1g **PROTEIN** 8g

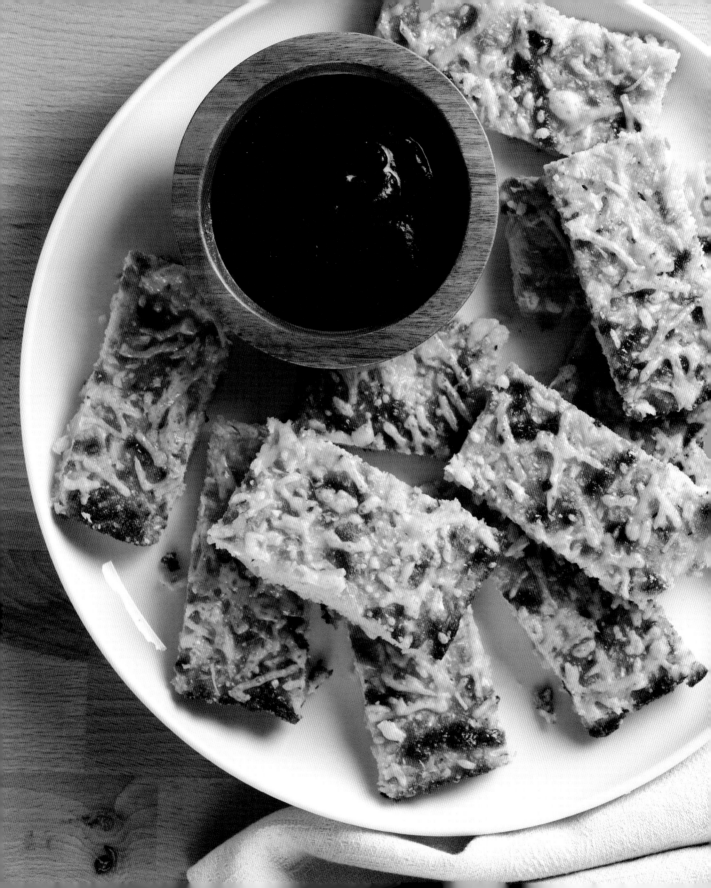

COCONUT CAULIFLOWER CREAM SOUP

MAKES 6 SERVINGS

1 tablespoon coconut oil

1 medium onion, chopped

1 tablespoon minced garlic

1 tablespoon minced fresh ginger

1 teaspoon salt

1 head cauliflower (1½ pounds), cut into florets

2 cans (about 13 ounces each) coconut milk, divided

1 cup water

1 teaspoon garam masala

½ teaspoon ground turmeric

Pinch of ground red pepper

Chopped fresh cilantro and/or hot chile oil (optional)

1 Heat coconut oil in large saucepan over medium-high heat. Add onion; cook and stir 5 minutes or until softened. Add garlic, ginger and salt; cook and stir 30 seconds.

2 Add cauliflower, 1 can of coconut milk, water, garam masala, turmeric and red pepper flakes. Reduce heat to medium; cover and simmer 20 minutes or until cauliflower is very tender.

3 Remove from heat. Blend soup with immersion blender until smooth. Return saucepan to medium heat; add 1 cup additional coconut milk. Cook and stir until heated through. Add additional coconut milk, if desired, to reach desired consistency. Garnish with cilantro.

NUTRIENTS PER SERVING (SERVING SIZE: ⅙ OF TOTAL RECIPE; ABOUT 1 CUP SOUP)

CALORIES 310   **TOTAL FAT** 29g   **CARBS** 11g   **NET CARBS** 8g   **DIETARY FIBER** 3g   **PROTEIN** 5g

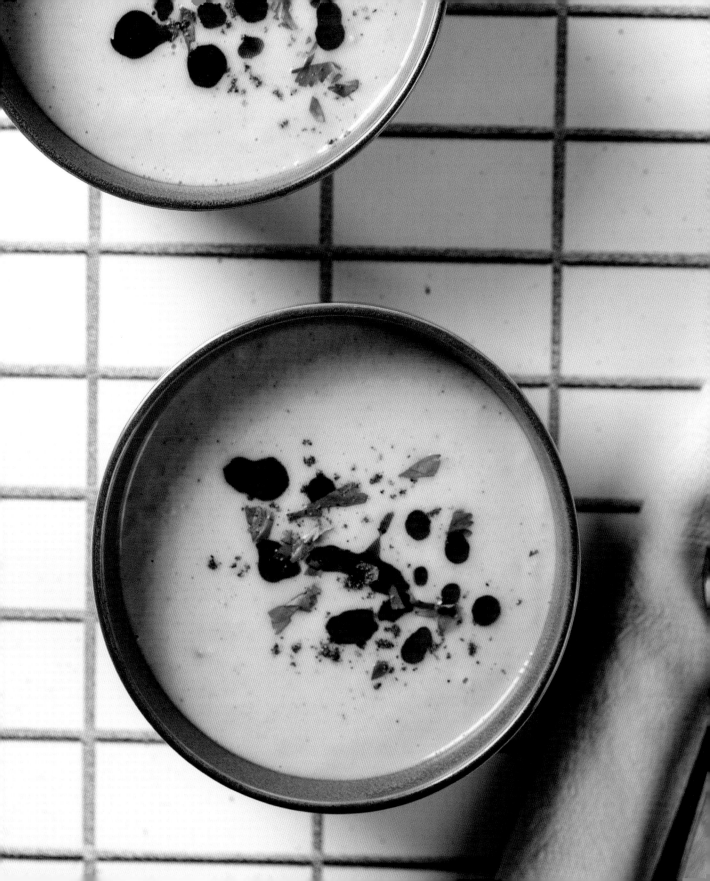

BUFFALO WINGS

MAKES 4 SERVINGS

1 cup hot pepper sauce

⅓ cup mild olive oil, plus additional for frying

½ teaspoon ground red pepper

½ teaspoon garlic powder

½ teaspoon Worcestershire sauce

⅛ teaspoon black pepper

1 pound chicken wings, tips discarded, separated at joints

Blue cheese dressing and celery sticks (optional)

1 Combine hot pepper sauce, ⅓ cup oil, red pepper, garlic powder, Worcestershire sauce and black pepper in small saucepan; cook over medium heat 20 minutes, stirring occasionally. Remove from heat; pour sauce into large bowl.

2 Heat 3 inches of oil in large saucepan over medium-high heat to 350°F; adjust heat to maintain temperature during cooking. Add wings; cook 10 minutes or until crispy. Drain on wire rack set over paper towels.

3 Transfer wings to bowl of sauce; toss to coat. Serve with blue cheese dressing and celery sticks, if desired.

NUTRIENTS PER SERVING (SERVING SIZE: ¼ OF CHICKEN WINGS)

CALORIES 320   **TOTAL FAT** 25g   **CARBS** 2g   **NET CARBS** 1g   **DIETARY FIBER** 1g   **PROTEIN** 20g

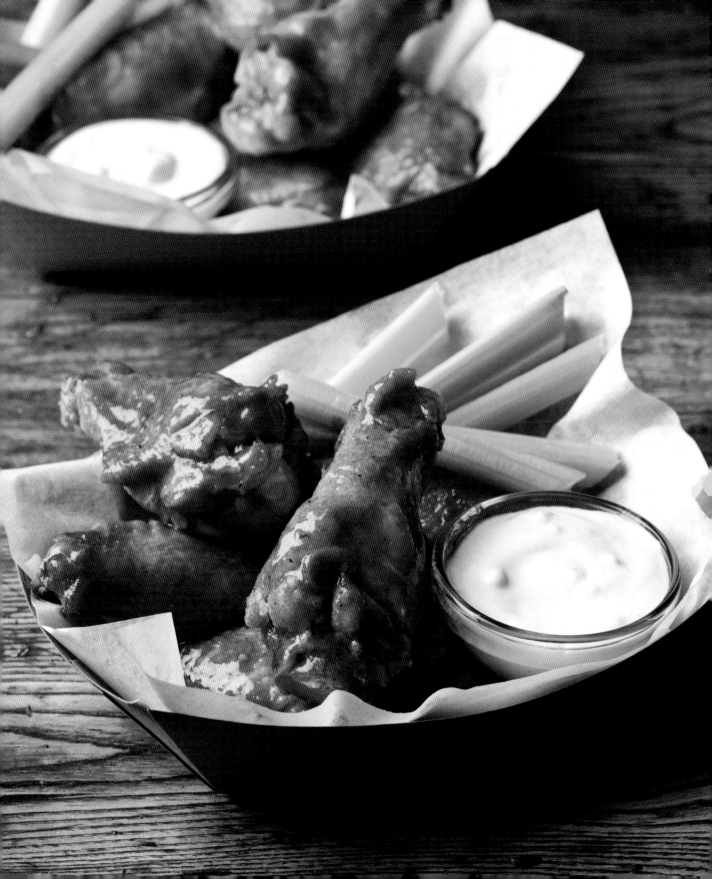

ROAST BEEF ROLL-UPS

MAKES 2 SERVINGS

2 tablespoons
   horseradish
   mayonnaise*

2 thin slices roast beef
   (1 ounce)

¼ cup crumbled blue
   cheese

¼ cup sliced red onion

*Or stir ½ teaspoon
horseradish into
2 tablespoons mayonnaise.*

1 Spread mayonnaise on roast beef slices. Sprinkle with blue cheese; layer with onion slices.

2 Roll up roast beef from short ends.

NUTRIENTS PER SERVING (SERVING SIZE: 1 ROLL-UP)

CALORIES 80   **TOTAL FAT** 5g   **CARBS** 2g   **NET CARBS** 1g   **DIETARY FIBER** 1g   **PROTEIN** 6g

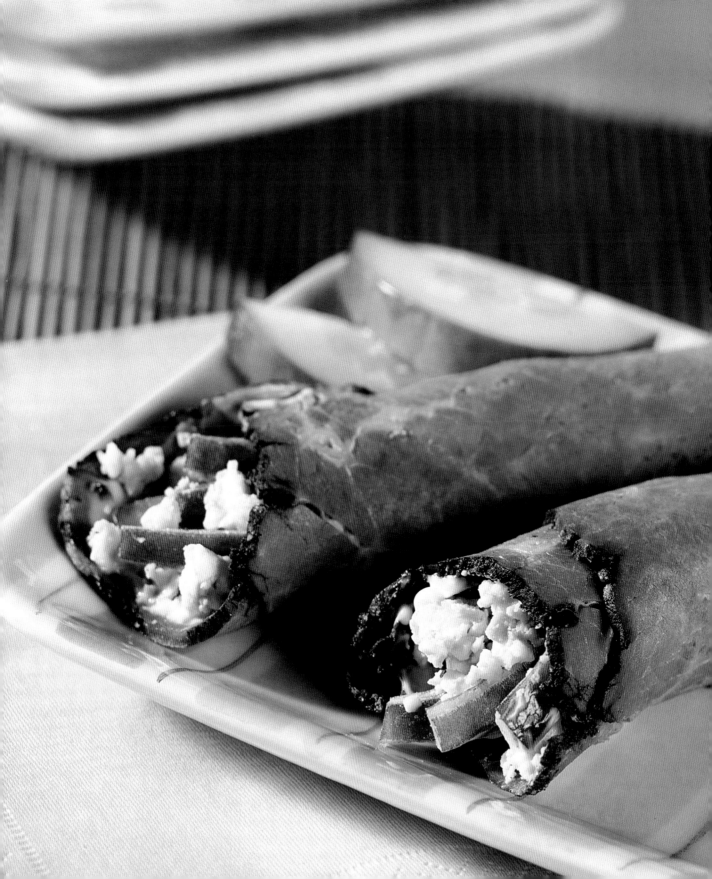

CRISPY CHEESE CHIPS

MAKES 8 SERVINGS

1½ cups (6 ounces) shredded mozzarella cheese*

½ cup grated Parmesan cheese

4 green onions, halved lengthwise and thinly sliced

1 teaspoon chili powder

1 teaspoon black pepper

Shred cheese using largest holes on box grater. If purchasing shredded cheese, look for the largest shreds available.

1 Place mozzarella in colander with large holes; shake to separate large shreds of cheese from smaller shreds; save smaller shreds for another use. Transfer large shreds of cheese to medium bowl; add Parmesan and toss to blend. Add green onions, chili powder and pepper; toss gently.

2 Line baking sheet with parchment paper. Spray medium nonstick skillet with nonstick cooking spray; heat over medium-high heat. Sprinkle about 1 tablespoon cheese mixture in single layer in skillet making lacy 2-inch circle. Cook 1 to 1½ minutes until cheese melts and turns golden brown. Immediately remove from skillet with thin spatula; cool completely on prepared baking sheet. Repeat with remaining cheese mixture.

NOTE

Cheese chips are extremely hot and pliable when they are first removed from pan but become crispy and chewy as they cool. To mold them into curls, drape them over a parchment-lined rolling pin while they're still hot.

NUTRIENTS PER SERVING (SERVING SIZE: 5 CHIPS)

CALORIES 88   **TOTAL FAT** 6g   **CARBS** 2g   **NET CARBS** 2g   **DIETARY FIBER** 0g   **PROTEIN** 7g

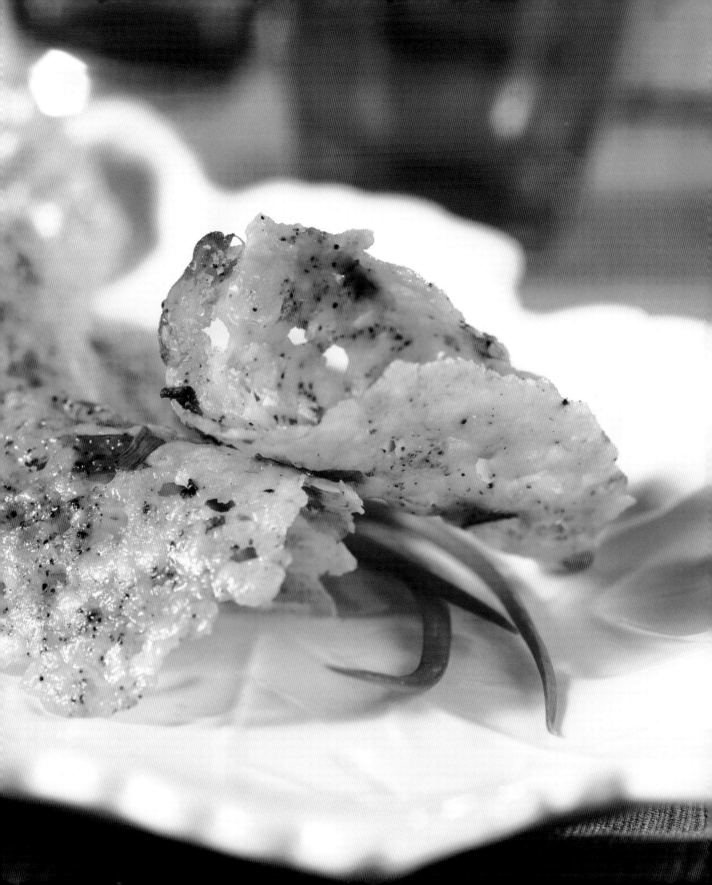

ROSEMARY NUT MIX

MAKES 32 SERVINGS

- 2 tablespoons butter
- 2 cups pecan halves
- 1 cup unsalted macadamia nuts
- 1 cup walnuts
- 1 teaspoon dried rosemary
- ½ teaspoon salt
- ¼ teaspoon red pepper flakes

1 Preheat oven to 300°F.

2 Melt butter in large saucepan over low heat. Stir in pecans, macadamia nuts and walnuts. Add rosemary, salt and red pepper flakes; cook and stir about 1 minute. Spread mixture on ungreased baking sheet.

3 Bake 8 to 10 minutes until nuts are fragrant and lightly browned, stirring occasionally. Cool completely on baking sheet on wire rack.

NUTRIENTS PER SERVING (SERVING SIZE: 2 TABLESPOONS MIX)

CALORIES 108 　　**TOTAL FAT** 11g 　　**CARBS** 2g 　　**NET CARBS** 1g 　　**DIETARY FIBER** 1g 　　**PROTEIN** 2g

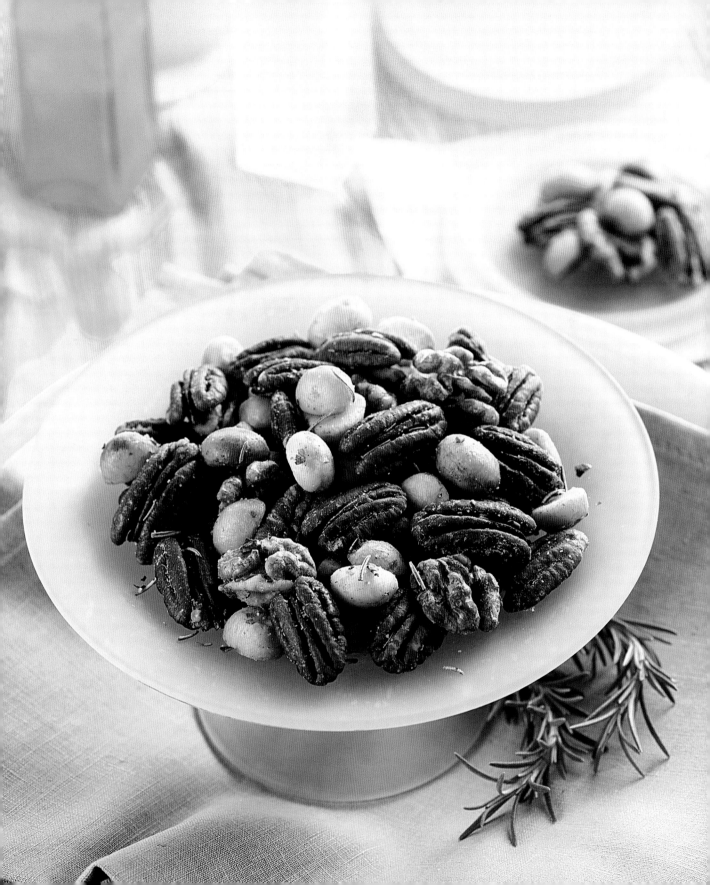

BELL PEPPER WEDGES
WITH HERBED GOAT CHEESE

MAKES 6 SERVINGS

2 small red bell peppers

1 log (4 ounces) plain goat cheese, softened

⅓ cup whipped cream cheese

2 tablespoons minced fresh chives

1 teaspoon minced fresh dill

1 Cut tops off of bell peppers; remove core and seeds. Cut each pepper into six wedges. Remove ribs, if necessary.

2 Combine goat cheese, cream cheese, chives and dill in small bowl; stir until well blended. Pipe or spread 1 tablespoon goat cheese mixture onto each pepper wedge.

NUTRIENTS PER SERVING (SERVING SIZE: 2 WEDGES)

CALORIES 110   **TOTAL FAT** 8g   **CARBS** 4g   **NET CARBS** 3g   **DIETARY FIBER** 1g   **PROTEIN** 5g

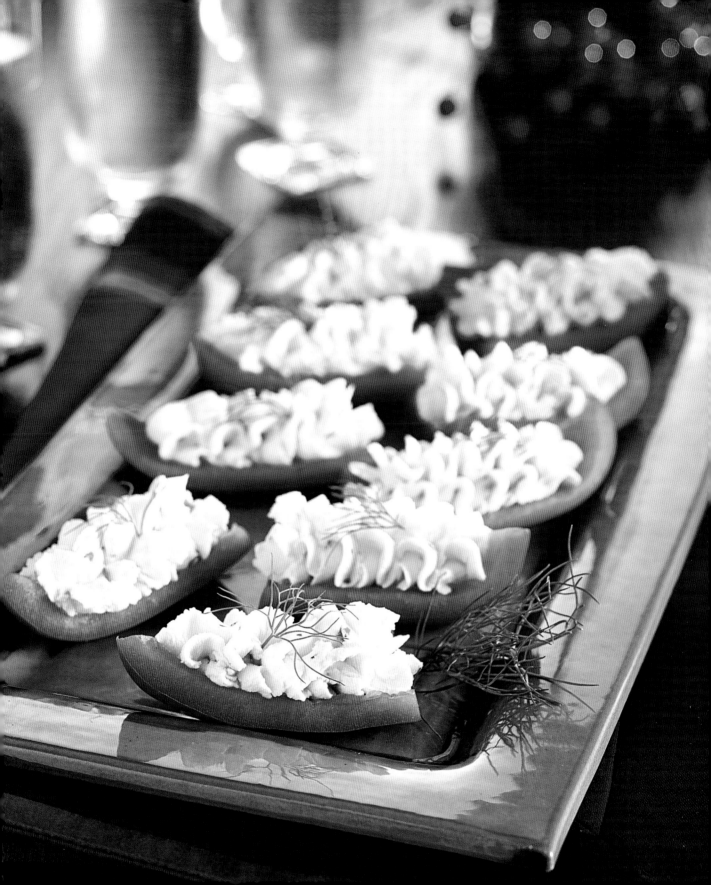

CREAM OF AVOCADO SOUP

MAKES 6 SERVINGS

3 medium avocados,
    cut into halves and
    pitted
  Lemon juice
½ cup vegetable broth,
    divided
2 eggs*
2 cups whole milk,
    divided
½ teaspoon salt
⅛ teaspoon white pepper
1½ cups sour cream,
    divided
  Black caviar and
    ground red pepper
    (optional)

Use clean, uncracked eggs.

1 Scoop out flesh of avocados leaving ¼-inch shell; set aside avocado flesh. Lightly sprinkle shells with lemon juice to prevent browning. Cover; refrigerate.

2 Process avocado flesh and ¼ cup broth in small batches in food processor or blender until smooth. Transfer to large bowl; set aside.

3 In top of double boiler, beat eggs with 1 cup milk. Heat slowly over hot, not boiling, water; stir until mixture is thick enough to coat back of spoon. Remove from heat; stir in remaining ¼ cup broth. Let stand at room temperature until cool.

4 Stir cooled egg mixture, salt and white pepper into avocado mixture. Mix in 1 cup plus 2 tablespoons sour cream, stirring until smooth. Add remaining 1 cup milk. Process soup in batches in food processor until smooth. Adjust seasonings. Cover and refrigerate until cold.

5 To serve, pour cold soup into avocado shells. Top each serving with 1 tablespoon sour cream. Garnish, if desired.

NUTRIENTS PER SERVING (SERVING SIZE: 1 FILLED AVOCADO HALF)

CALORIES 360   **TOTAL FAT** 31g   **CARBS** 15g   **NET CARBS** 8g   **DIETARY FIBER** 7g   **PROTEIN** 9g

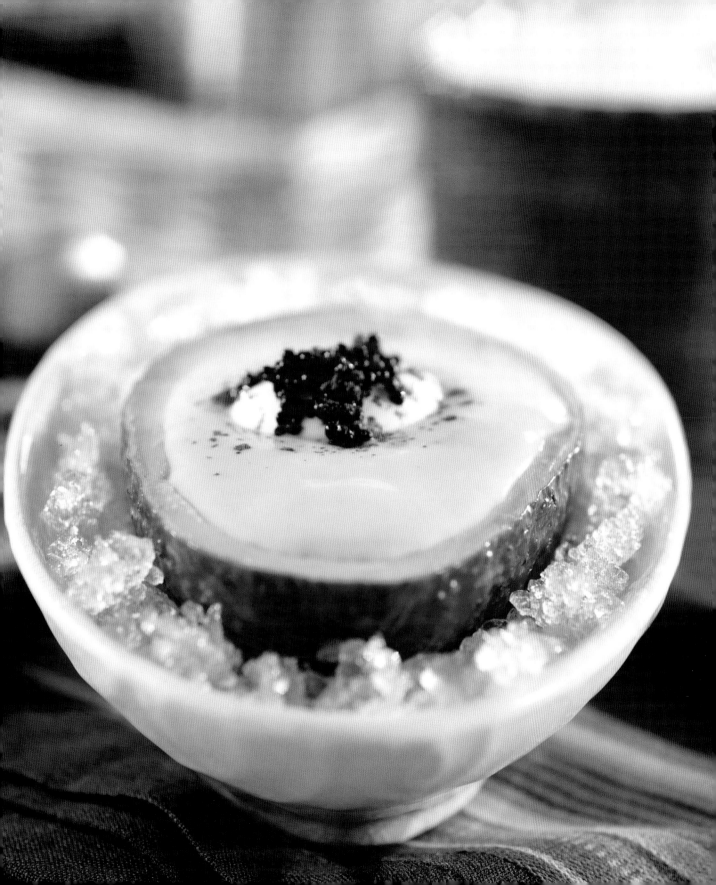

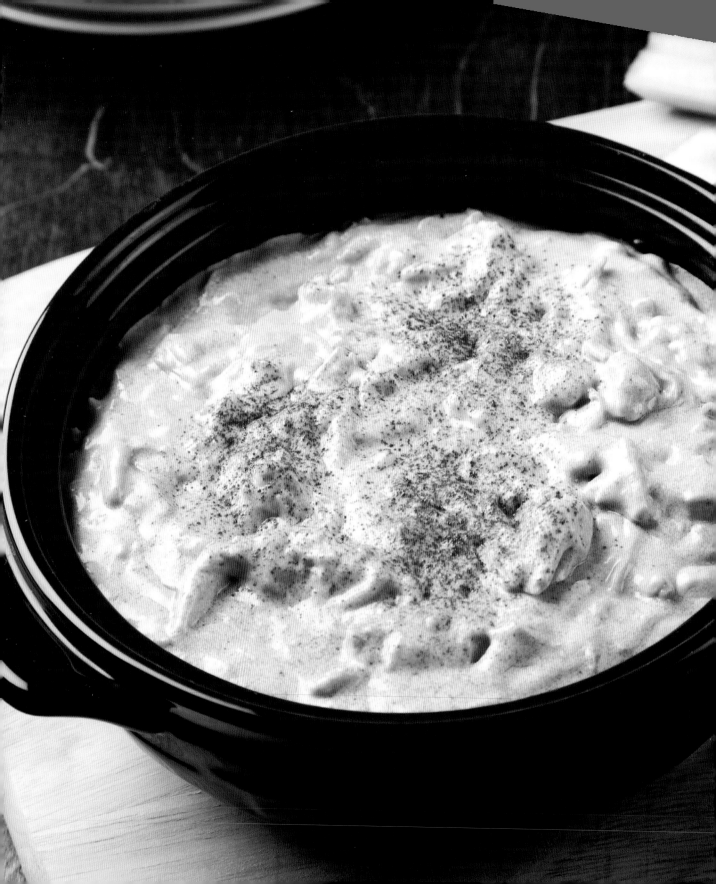

DIPS
AND SPREADS

BUFFALO CHICKEN DIP
MAKES 5 CUPS (20 SERVINGS)

2 packages (8 ounces each) cream cheese, softened and cut into pieces

1 jar (12 ounces) buffalo wing sauce

1 cup keto ranch dressing

2 cups shredded cooked chicken (from 1 pound boneless skinless chicken breasts)

2 cups (8 ounces) shredded Cheddar cheese

Paprika (optional)

Celery sticks

1 Combine cream cheese, wing sauce and ranch dressing in large saucepan; cook over medium-low heat 7 to 10 minutes or until cream cheese is melted and mixture is smooth, whisking frequently.

2 Combine chicken and Cheddar cheese in large bowl. Add cream cheese mixture; stir until well blended. Pour into serving bowl; sprinkle with paprika, if desired. Serve warm with celery sticks.

NUTRIENTS PER SERVING (SERVING SIZE: ¼ CUP)

CALORIES	TOTAL FAT	CARBS	NET CARBS	DIETARY FIBER	PROTEIN
190	15g	3g	3g	0g	9g

BACON & ONION CHEESE BALL

MAKES 20 SERVINGS

1 package (8 ounces) cream cheese, softened

½ cup sour cream

½ cup crumbled cooked bacon

½ cup chopped green onions, plus additional for garnish

¼ cup crumbled blue cheese

Celery sticks

1 Whisk cream cheese, sour cream, bacon, ½ cup green onions and blue cheese in large bowl until well blended. Shape mixture into a ball. Wrap in plastic wrap; refrigerate at least 1 hour.

2 Place cheese ball on serving plate. Garnish with additional green onions. Serve with celery sticks.

NUTRIENTS PER SERVING (SERVING SIZE: 2 TABLESPOONS)

CALORIES 77   TOTAL FAT 6g   CARBS 2g   NET CARBS 1g   DIETARY FIBER 1g   PROTEIN 4g

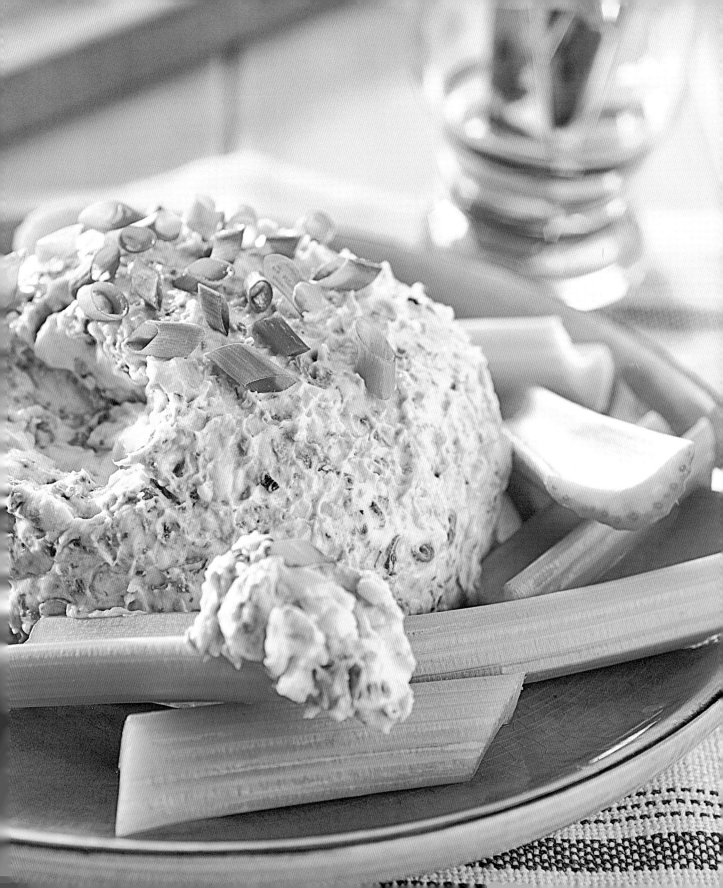

HOT CRAB DIP

MAKES 14 SERVINGS

4 ounces cream cheese, softened

½ cup sour cream

2 tablespoons mayonnaise

¾ teaspoon seasoned salt

¼ teaspoon paprika, plus additional for garnish

2 cans (6 ounces each) crabmeat, drained and flaked

½ cup (2 ounces) shredded mozzarella cheese

2 tablespoons minced onion

2 tablespoons finely chopped green bell pepper*

Chopped fresh parsley (optional)

Celery sticks

For a spicier dip, substitute 1 tablespoon minced jalapeño pepper for the bell pepper.

1 Preheat oven to 350°F.

2 Combine cream cheese, sour cream, mayonnaise, seasoned salt and ¼ teaspoon paprika in medium bowl; stir until well blended and smooth. Add crabmeat, cheese, onion and bell pepper; stir until blended. Spread in small (1-quart) shallow baking dish.

3 Bake 15 to 20 minutes or until bubbly and top is beginning to brown. Garnish with additional paprika and parsley; serve with celery sticks.

NUTRIENTS PER SERVING (SERVING SIZE: ¼ CUP)

CALORIES 110   **TOTAL FAT** 9g   **CARBS** 2g   **NET CARBS** 2g   **DIETARY FIBER** 0g   **PROTEIN** 6g

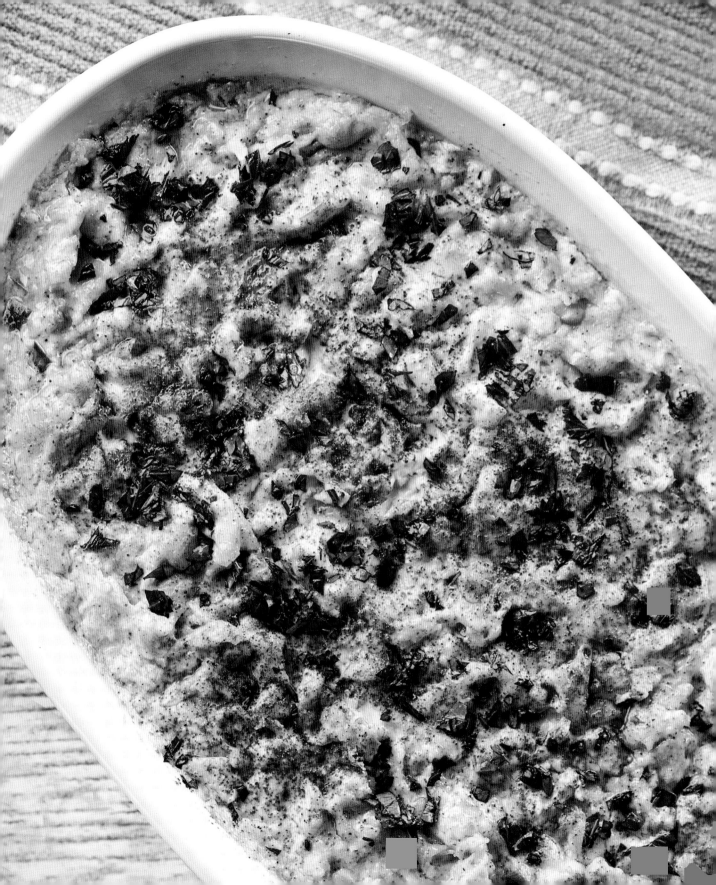

AVOCADO SALSA

MAKES 4 CUPS (32 SERVINGS)

1 medium avocado, diced

1 cup chopped onion

1 cup chopped peeled seeded cucumber

1 Anaheim pepper, seeded and chopped

½ cup chopped fresh tomato

2 tablespoons chopped fresh cilantro, plus additional for garnish

½ teaspoon salt

¼ teaspoon hot pepper sauce

1 Combine avocado, onion, cucumber, Anaheim pepper, tomato, 2 tablespoons cilantro, salt and hot pepper sauce in medium bowl; mix gently.

2 Cover and refrigerate at least 1 hour before serving. Garnish with additional cilantro.

NUTRIENTS PER SERVING (SERVING SIZE: 2 TABLESPOONS)

CALORIES 13   **TOTAL FAT** 1g   **CARBS** 1g   **NET CARBS** 0g   **DIETARY FIBER** 1g   **PROTEIN** 1g

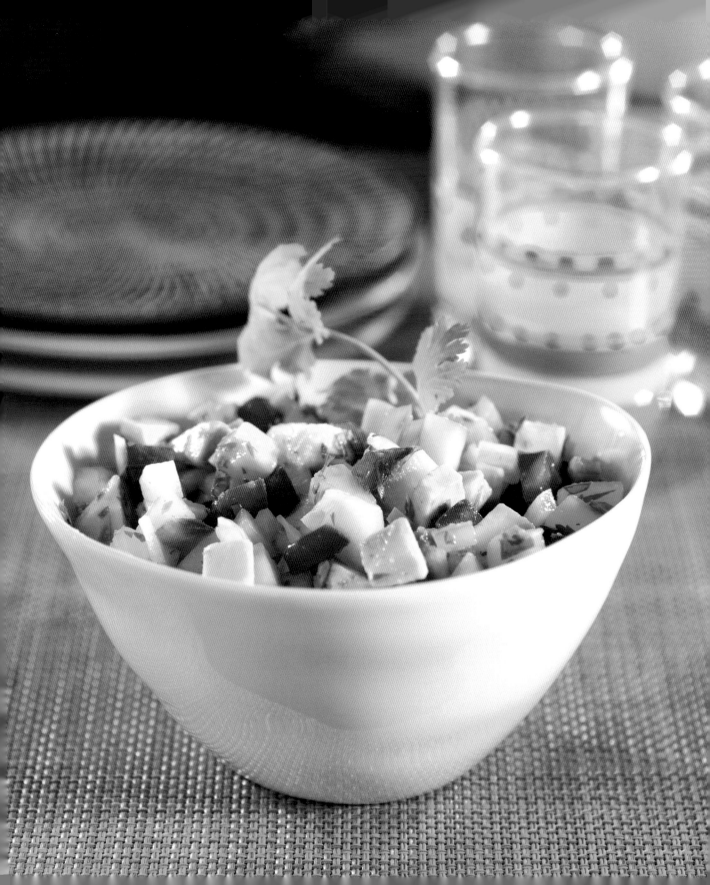

SMOKED SALMON SPREAD

MAKES 1½ CUPS (12 SERVINGS)

1 package (8 ounces) cream cheese, softened

3 ounces smoked salmon (lox), coarsely chopped

2 tablespoons fresh lemon juice

1 tablespoon chopped fresh dill

1 tablespoon capers

Cucumber slices

1 Combine cream cheese, salmon, lemon juice, dill and capers in small bowl; mix well.

2 Serve immediately or cover and refrigerate up to 3 days. Serve with cucumber slices.

TIP ||||||||||||||||||||||||||||||||||||||||||||||||||||||||||||||||||||||||||||||||||||||||

This savory spread tastes like a mix of favorite bagel toppings. Try it on a piece of toasted keto bread (page 180) or a keto everything bagel (page 98) for breakfast.

NUTRIENTS PER SERVING (SERVING SIZE: 2 TABLESPOONS)

CALORIES 90   TOTAL FAT 8g   CARBS 1g   NET CARBS 1g   DIETARY FIBER 0g   PROTEIN 4g

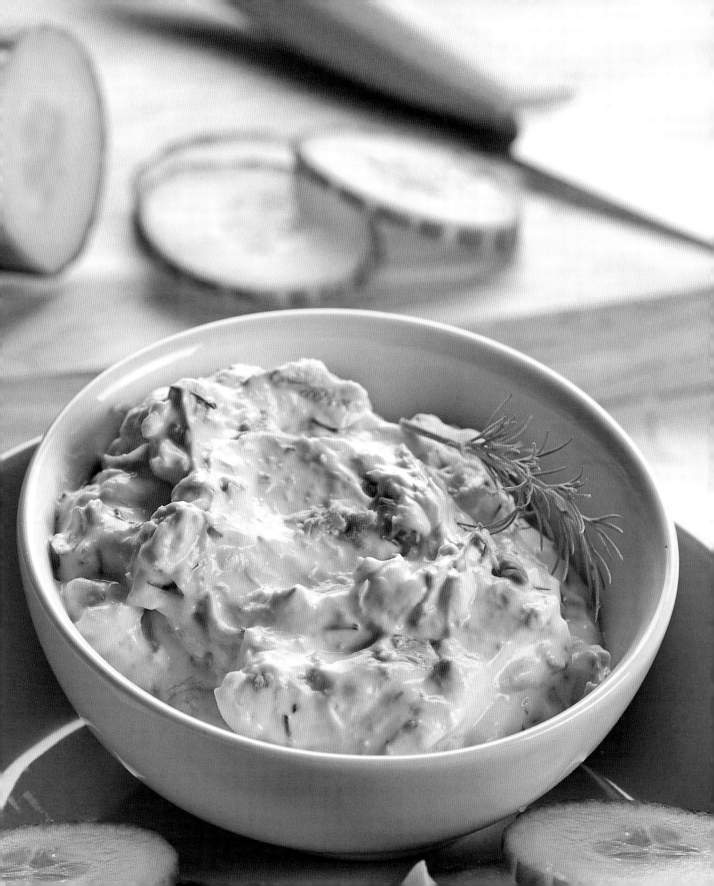

BAGNA CAUDA
MAKES 1½ CUPS (12 SERVINGS)

¾ cup olive oil

6 tablespoons butter, softened

12 anchovy fillets, drained

6 cloves garlic, peeled

⅛ teaspoon red pepper flakes

Fresh vegetables for dipping: endive spears, cauliflower florets, cucumber sticks, zucchini sticks and/or red bell pepper strips

1 Combine oil, butter, anchovies, garlic and red pepper flakes in food processor; process until smooth.

2 Pour mixture into small saucepan. Cook over medium-low heat until warm, stirring frequently. Serve with vegetables for dipping.

TIP ||||||||||||||||||||||||||||||||||||||||||||||||||||||||||||||||||||||||||||||||||||||||||||||||||||

Bagna cauda is a warm Italian dip similar to fondue. The name means "warm bath" in Italian.

NUTRIENTS PER SERVING (SERVING SIZE: 2 TABLESPOONS)

CALORIES 220   TOTAL FAT 24g   CARBS 1g   NET CARBS 1g   DIETARY FIBER 0g   PROTEIN 2g

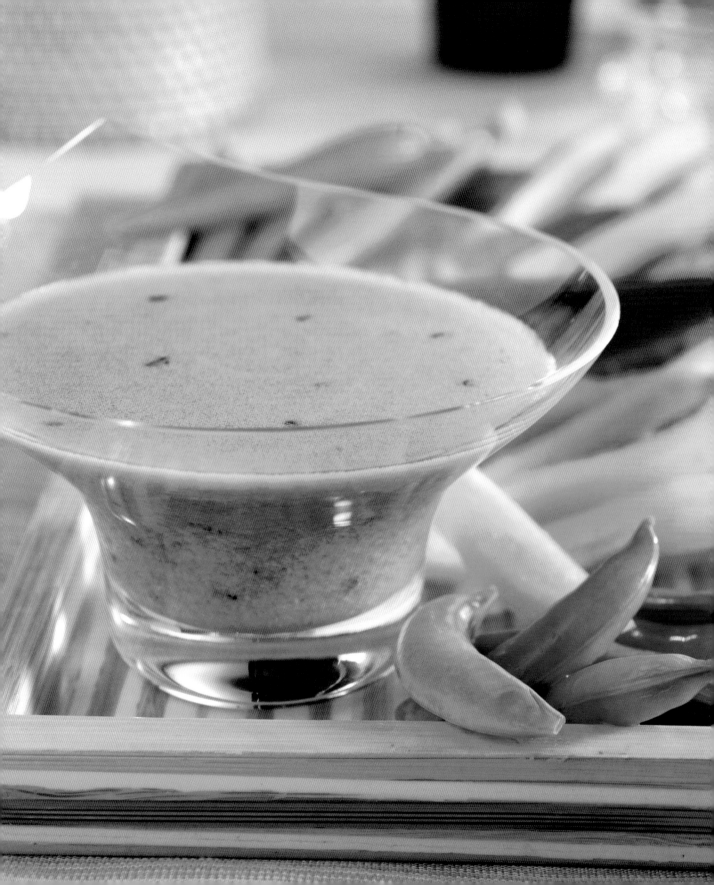

SPINACH, CRAB AND ARTICHOKE DIP

MAKES 2½ CUPS (10 SERVINGS)

1 can (6 ounces) crabmeat, drained and shredded

1 package (10 ounces) frozen chopped spinach, thawed and squeezed nearly dry

1 package (8 ounces) Neufchâtel cheese or regular cream cheese, softened

1 jar (about 6 ounces) marinated artichoke hearts, drained and finely chopped

¼ teaspoon hot pepper sauce

Keto crackers and/or bell pepper strips (optional)

Slow Cooker Directions

1 Pick out and discard any shell or cartilage from crabmeat.

2 Combine crabmeat, spinach, cream cheese, artichokes and hot pepper sauce in 1½-quart slow cooker. Cover; cook on HIGH 1½ to 2 hours or until heated through, stirring after 1 hour. Serve with keto crackers or bell pepper strips, if desired.

NUTRIENTS PER SERVING (SERVING SIZE: ¼ CUP)

| CALORIES 99 | TOTAL FAT 7g | CARBS 3g | NET CARBS 2g | DIETARY FIBER 1g | PROTEIN 6g |

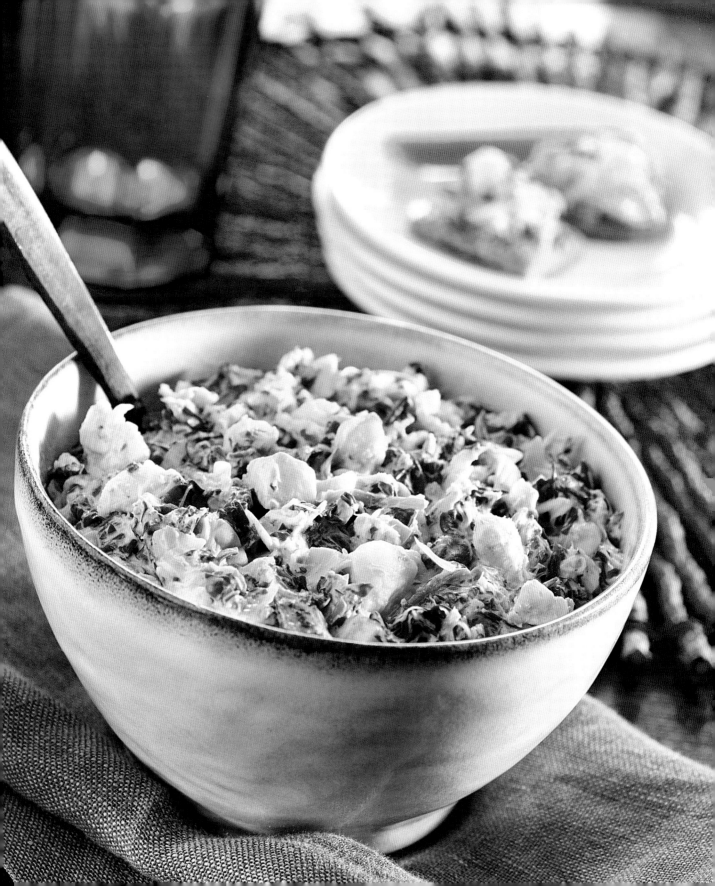

ROASTED RED PEPPER DIP

MAKES 2 CUPS (ABOUT 16 SERVINGS)

2 jars (12 ounces each) roasted red peppers in water, drained

1 cup crumbled feta cheese

¼ cup chopped fresh basil

¼ cup sour cream

3 tablespoons Worcestershire sauce

4 cloves garlic

Bell pepper sticks and/or broccoli florets

1 Place roasted red peppers in food processor or blender; process until coarsely chopped. Add cheese, basil, sour cream, Worcestershire sauce and garlic; process until smooth and well blended. Cover and refrigerate at least 2 hours or until cold.

2 Serve with vegetables for dipping.

NUTRIENTS PER SERVING (SERVING SIZE: 2 TABLESPOONS)

CALORIES 40 **TOTAL FAT** 3g **CARBS** 2g **NET CARBS** 2g **DIETARY FIBER** 0g **PROTEIN** 2g

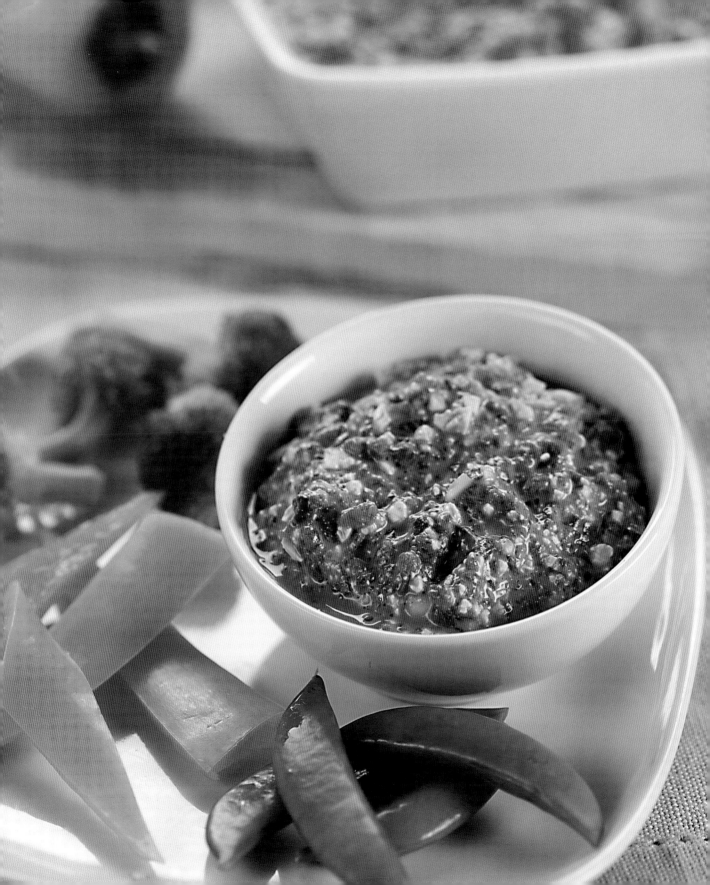

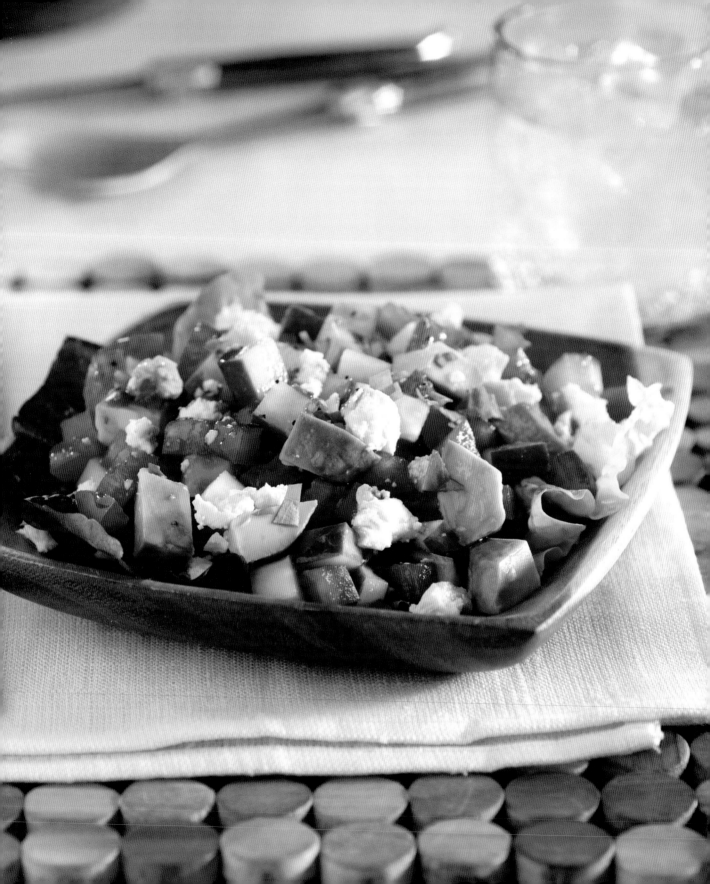

SALADS
AND VEGETABLES

TOMATO, AVOCADO AND CUCUMBER SALAD
MAKES 4 SERVINGS

1½ tablespoons extra virgin olive oil

1 tablespoon balsamic vinegar

1 clove garlic, minced

¼ teaspoon salt

¼ teaspoon black pepper

2 cups diced seeded plum tomatoes

1 ripe avocado, diced (½-inch pieces)

½ cup chopped cucumber

⅓ cup crumbled feta cheese

Lettuce leaves (optional)

Chopped fresh basil (optional)

1 Whisk oil, vinegar, garlic, salt and pepper in medium bowl. Add tomatoes and avocado; toss gently to coat. Stir in cucumber and feta.

2 Arrange lettuce leaves on serving plates; top with salad and sprinkle with basil, if desired.

NUTRIENTS PER SERVING (SERVING SIZE: ABOUT ¾ CUP)

CALORIES 138 **TOTAL FAT** 11g **CARBS** 7g **NET CARBS** 5g **DIETARY FIBER** 2g **PROTEIN** 4g

GARBAGE SALAD
MAKES 4 SERVINGS

DRESSING

- ⅓ cup red wine vinegar
- 2 cloves garlic, minced
- 1 teaspoon Italian seasoning
- ¼ teaspoon salt
- ¼ teaspoon black pepper
- ⅓ cup olive oil

SALAD

- 1 package (5 ounces) spring mix
- 5 leaves romaine lettuce, chopped
- 1 small cucumber, diced
- 2 small plum tomatoes, diced
- ½ red onion, thinly sliced
- ¼ cup pitted kalamata olives
- 4 radishes, thinly sliced
- 4 ounces thinly sliced Genoa salami, cut into ¼-inch strips
- 4 ounces provolone cheese, cut into ¼-inch strips
- ¼ cup grated Parmesan cheese

1 For dressing, whisk vinegar, garlic, Italian seasoning, salt and pepper in small bowl until blended. Slowly whisk in oil in thin steady stream until well blended.

2 Combine spring mix, romaine, cucumber, tomatoes, onion, olives and radishes in large bowl. Add half of dressing; toss gently to coat. Top with salami and provolone; sprinkle with Parmesan. Serve with remaining dressing.

NUTRIENTS PER SERVING (SERVING SIZE: ¼ OF TOTAL RECIPE)

CALORIES 420 **TOTAL FAT** 35g **CARBS** 10g **NET CARBS** 7g **DIETARY FIBER** 3g **PROTEIN** 19g

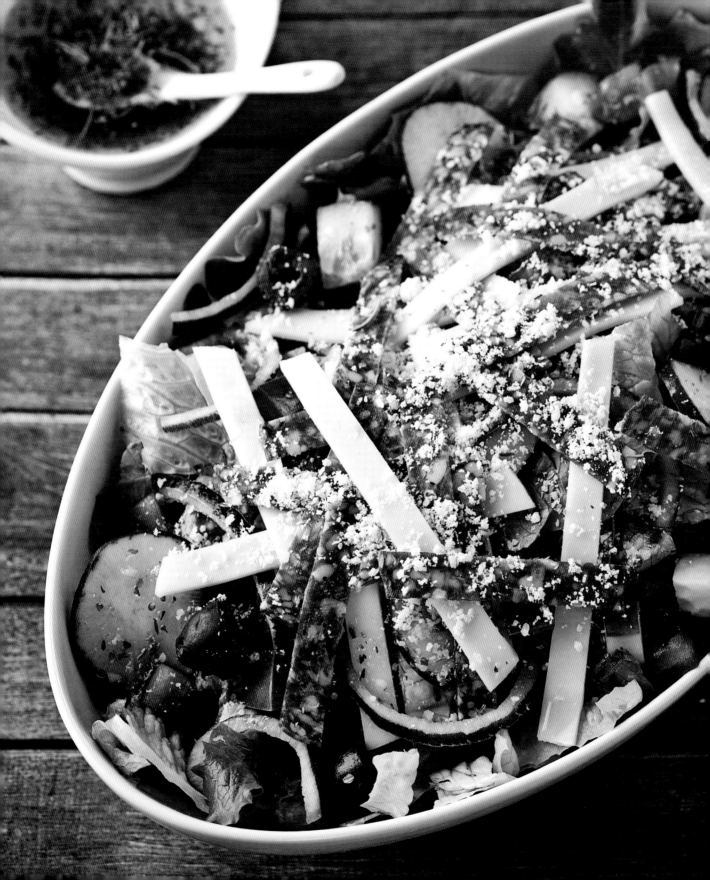

COLORFUL COLESLAW

MAKES 8 SERVINGS

¼ head green cabbage, shredded or thinly sliced

¼ head red cabbage, shredded or thinly sliced

1 small yellow or orange bell pepper, thinly sliced

1 small jicama, peeled and julienned

¼ cup thinly sliced green onions

2 tablespoons chopped fresh cilantro

¼ cup mild olive oil

¼ cup fresh lime juice

1 teaspoon salt

⅛ teaspoon black pepper

1 Combine cabbage, bell pepper, jicama, green onions and cilantro in large bowl.

2 Whisk oil, lime juice, salt and black pepper in small bowl until well blended. Pour over vegetables; toss to coat. Cover and refrigerate 2 to 6 hours for flavors to blend.

NUTRIENTS PER SERVING (SERVING SIZE: ⅛ OF TOTAL RECIPE)

CALORIES 200 **TOTAL FAT** 14g **CARBS** 19g **NET CARBS** 11g **DIETARY FIBER** 8g **PROTEIN** 3g

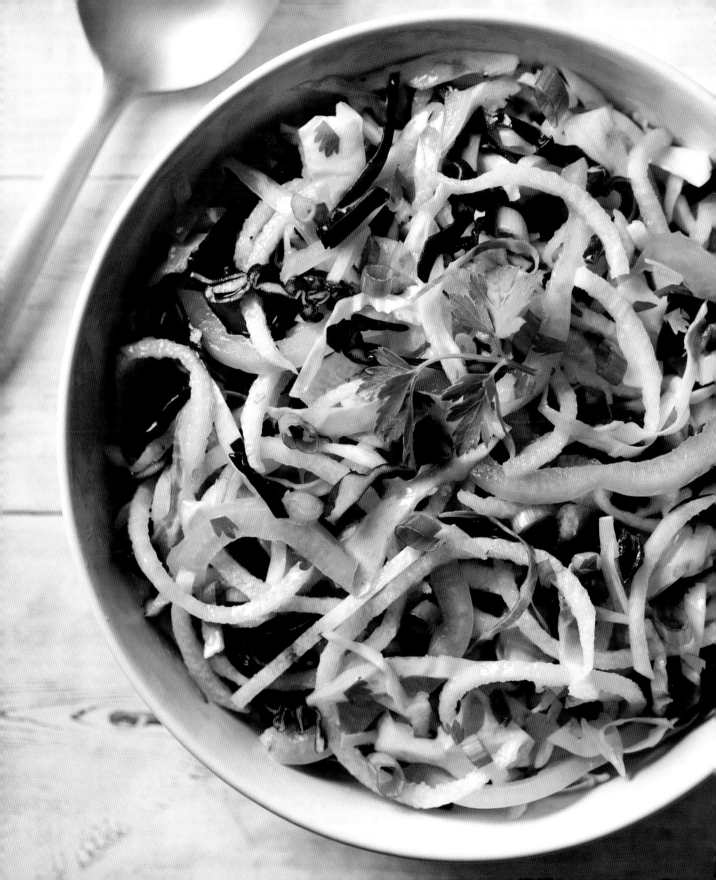

CHICKEN SALAD BOWL

MAKES 4 SERVINGS

CHICKEN

- 1 **pound boneless skinless chicken breasts**
- 3 **tablespoons olive oil, divided**
- 1 **teaspoon salt**
- 1 **teaspoon dried oregano**
- 1 **teaspoon paprika**
- ½ **teaspoon black pepper**
- 1 **clove garlic, minced**

SALAD AND DRESSING

- ⅓ **cup olive oil**
- 3 **tablespoons red wine vinegar**
- 1 **clove garlic, minced**

   Salt and black pepper
- 1 **cup grape tomatoes, halved**
- 1 **cucumber, halved crosswise and cut into sticks**
- 1 **red bell pepper, sliced**
- 2 **avocados, thinly sliced**
- 2 **radishes, thinly sliced**

   Leaf lettuce and arugula

   Black and white sesame seeds (optional)

1 Pound chicken to 1-inch thickness between sheets of plastic wrap. Combine 1 tablespoon oil, salt, oregano, paprika, black pepper and 1 clove garlic in small bowl. Sprinkle over both sides of chicken; pat to adhere spices to chicken.

2 Heat remaining 2 tablespoons oil in large skillet over medium-high heat. Add chicken; cook 8 to 10 minutes or until cooked through (165°F), turning once.

3 For dressing, whisk ⅓ cup oil, vinegar and 1 clove garlic in small bowl. Season to taste with salt and black pepper.

4 Place tomatoes, cucumber, bell pepper, avocados, radishes, lettuce and arugula in serving bowls; drizzle with dressing. Slice chicken and place on salads. Sprinkle with sesame seeds, if desired.

TIP

If your chicken is particularly large, cut it in half crosswise, making two thinner pieces. This will help it cook quicker and more evenly.

NUTRIENTS PER SERVING (SERVING SIZE: ¼ OF TOTAL RECIPE)

| **CALORIES** 570 | **TOTAL FAT** 44g | **CARBS** 18g | **NET CARBS** 9g | **DIETARY FIBER** 9g | **PROTEIN** 30g |

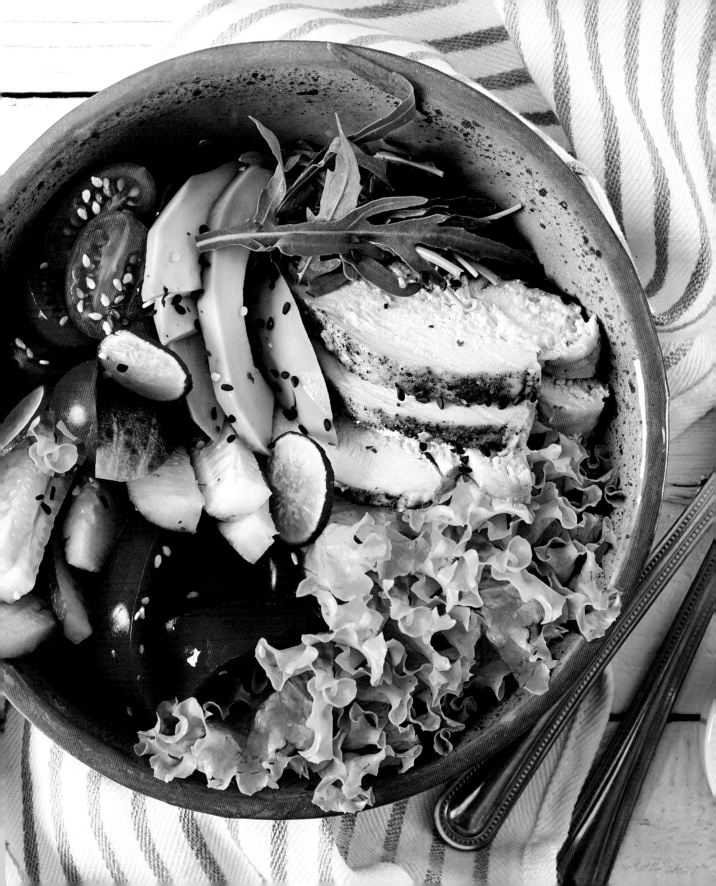

GREEK SALAD

MAKES 6 SERVINGS

SALAD

3 medium tomatoes, cut into 8 wedges each

1 green bell pepper, cut into 1-inch pieces

½ English cucumber (8 to 10 inches), quartered lengthwise and sliced crosswise

½ red onion, thinly sliced

½ cup pitted kalamata olives

1 block (8 ounces) feta cheese, cut into ½-inch cubes

Chopped fresh parsley

DRESSING

6 tablespoons extra virgin olive oil

3 tablespoons red wine vinegar

1 to 2 cloves garlic, minced

¾ teaspoon dried oregano

¾ teaspoon salt

¼ teaspoon black pepper

1 Combine tomatoes, bell pepper, cucumber, onion and olives in large bowl. Top with feta.

2 For dressing, whisk oil, vinegar, garlic, oregano, salt and pepper in medium bowl until well blended. Pour over salad; stir gently to coat. Sprinkle with parsley.

NUTRIENTS PER SERVING (SERVING SIZE: ⅙ OF TOTAL RECIPE)

CALORIES 233   **TOTAL FAT** 21g   **CARBS** 7g   **NET CARBS** 6g   **DIETARY FIBER** 1g   **PROTEIN** 8g

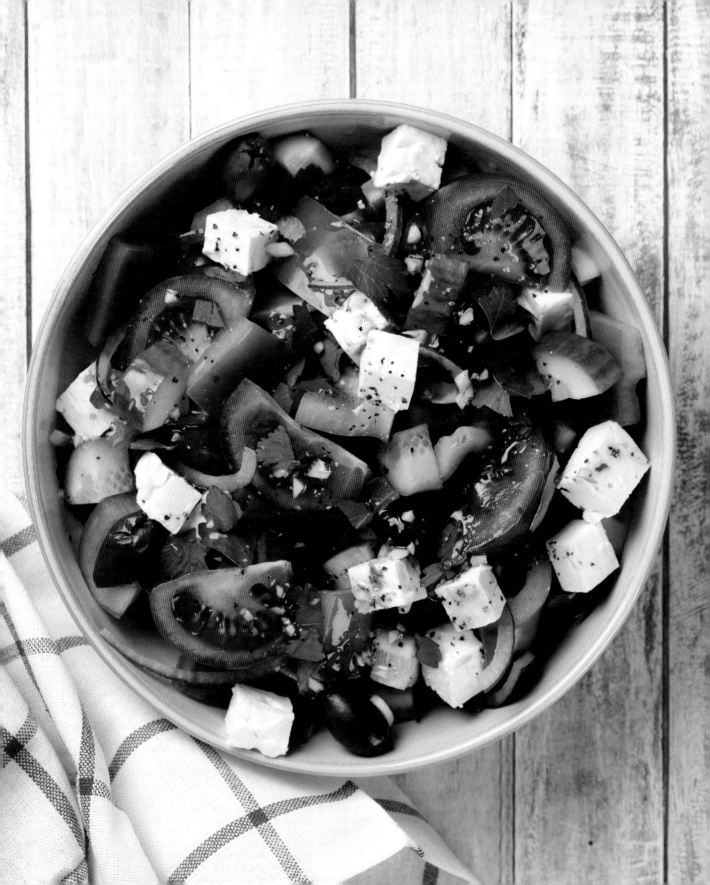

MASHED CAULIFLOWER

MAKES 6 SERVINGS

2 heads cauliflower
1 tablespoon butter
1 tablespoon half-and-half or whipping cream or as needed
Salt

1 Break cauliflower into equal-size florets. Place in large saucepan in about 2 inches of water. Simmer over medium heat 20 to 25 minutes or until cauliflower is very tender and falling apart. (Check occasionally to make sure there is enough water to prevent burning; add water if necessary.) Drain well.

2 Place cauliflower in food processor or blender. Process until almost smooth. Add butter; process until smooth, adding half-and-half as needed to reach desired consistency. Season with salt to taste.

NUTRIENTS PER SERVING (SERVING SIZE: ½ CUP)

CALORIES 54   **TOTAL FAT** 2g   **CARBS** 7g   **NET CARBS** 4g   **DIETARY FIBER** 3g   **PROTEIN** 3g

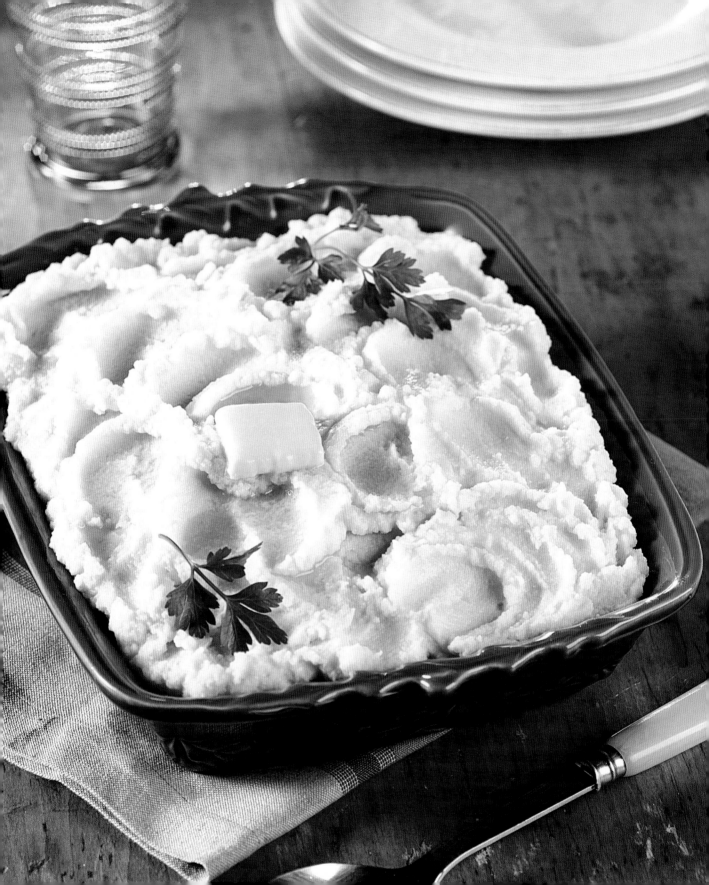

MEDITERRANEAN STEAK SALAD

MAKES 4 SERVINGS

STEAK

- 2 tablespoons olive oil
- 2 teaspoons salt
- 2 teaspoons dried oregano
- 2 teaspoons paprika
- 1 teaspoon black pepper
- 1 clove garlic, minced
- 4 sirloin steaks (about 8 ounces each)

SALAD AND DRESSING

- ⅓ cup olive oil
- 3 tablespoons red wine vinegar
- 1 clove garlic, minced
- ¾ teaspoon dried oregano
- ¾ teaspoon salt
- ¼ teaspoon black pepper
- 4 cups assorted mixed greens
- 2 medium tomatoes, cut into wedges
- ½ red onion, thinly sliced
- ½ cup pitted kalamata olives
- 4 ounces feta cheese, cut into cubes

1 Combine 2 tablespoons oil, 2 teaspoons salt, 2 teaspoons oregano, paprika, 1 teaspoon black pepper and 1 clove garlic in large bowl. Add steak; toss until well coated.

2 Oil grid. Prepare grill for direct cooking. Cook steak, covered, over medium-high heat about 6 minutes per side for medium or to desired doneness.

3 For dressing, whisk ⅓ cup oil, vinegar, 1 clove garlic, ¾ teaspoon oregano, ¾ teaspoon salt and ¼ teaspoon pepper in medium bowl.

4 Divide greens among four plates. Top with tomatoes, onion, olives, cheese and steak. Drizzle with dressing.

NUTRIENTS PER SERVING (SERVING SIZE: ¼ OF TOTAL RECIPE)

CALORIES 580   **TOTAL FAT** 40g   **CARBS** 9g   **NET CARBS** 7g   **DIETARY FIBER** 2g   **PROTEIN** 49g

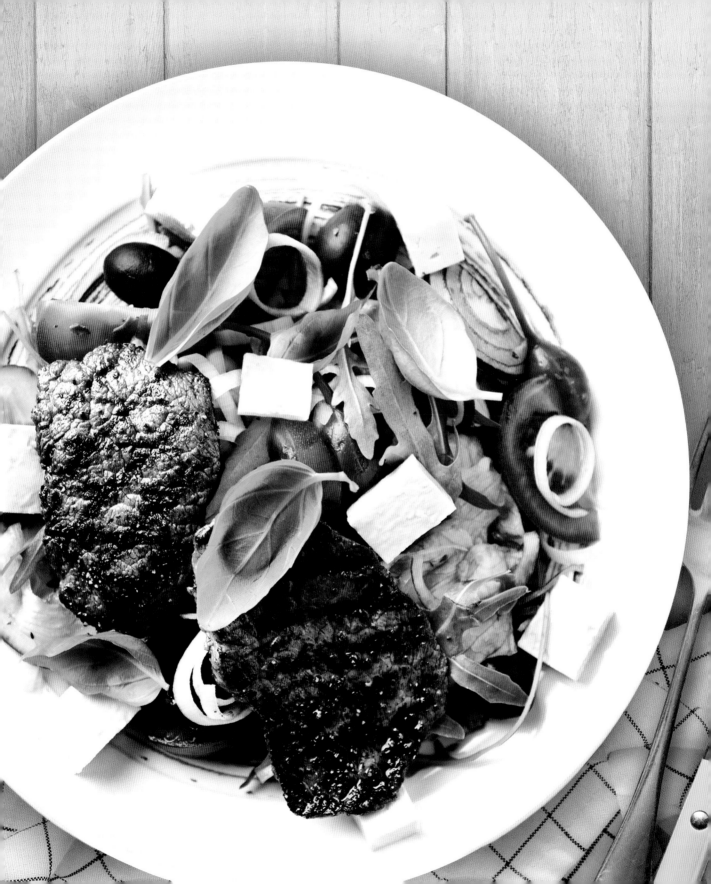

BROCCOLI ITALIAN STYLE

MAKES 4 SERVINGS

1¼ pounds fresh broccoli crowns

Salt and black pepper

2 tablespoons lemon juice

1 teaspoon extra virgin olive oil

1 clove garlic, minced

1 teaspoon chopped fresh Italian parsley

1 Trim broccoli, discarding tough stems. Cut broccoli into florets with 2-inch stems. Peel remaining stems; cut into ½-inch slices.

2 Bring 4 cups water to a boil in large saucepan over medium-high heat. Stir in 1 teaspoon salt. Add broccoli; return to a boil. Cook 3 to 5 minutes or until broccoli is tender. Drain; transfer to serving dish.

3 Combine lemon juice, oil, garlic and parsley in small bowl. Pour over broccoli; toss to coat. Cover and let stand 1 hour before serving to allow flavors to blend. Season with salt and pepper to taste. Serve at room temperature.

NUTRIENTS PER SERVING (SERVING SIZE: ¼ OF TOTAL RECIPE)

CALORIES 44   **TOTAL FAT** 2g   **CARBS** 7g   **NET CARBS** 4g   **DIETARY FIBER** 3g   **PROTEIN** 3g

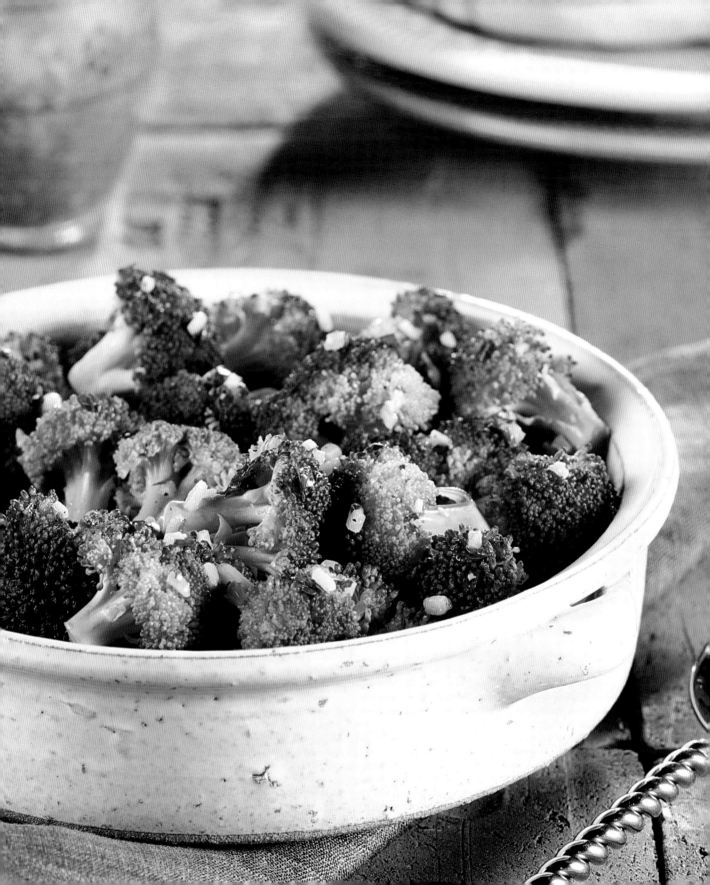

EGGPLANT ROLLS

MAKES 6 APPETIZER SERVINGS

1 large eggplant (about 1¼ pounds)

3 tablespoons extra virgin olive oil

Salt and black pepper

1 cup ricotta cheese

½ cup grated Asiago cheese

¼ cup julienned or chopped oil-packed sun-dried tomatoes

¼ cup chopped fresh basil or Italian parsley

⅛ teaspoon red pepper flakes

1 Preheat broiler. Trim stem end from eggplant; discard. Peel eggplant, if desired. Cut eggplant lengthwise into 6 slices about ¼ inch thick. Brush both sides of eggplant slices with oil; sprinkle with salt and black pepper. Place on rack of broiler pan or on wire rack set on baking sheet.

2 Broil 4 inches from heat 4 to 5 minutes per side or until golden brown and slightly softened. Cool to room temperature.

3 Combine ricotta, Asiago, sun-dried tomatoes, basil and red pepper flakes in small bowl; mix well. Spread mixture evenly over eggplant slices. Roll up and cut each roll in half crosswise. Arrange rolls, seam side down, on serving platter. Serve warm or at room temperature.

NUTRIENTS PER SERVING (SERVING SIZE: 1 ROLL)

CALORIES 200   **TOTAL FAT** 15g   **CARBS** 9g   **NET CARBS** 6g   **DIETARY FIBER** 3g   **PROTEIN** 8g

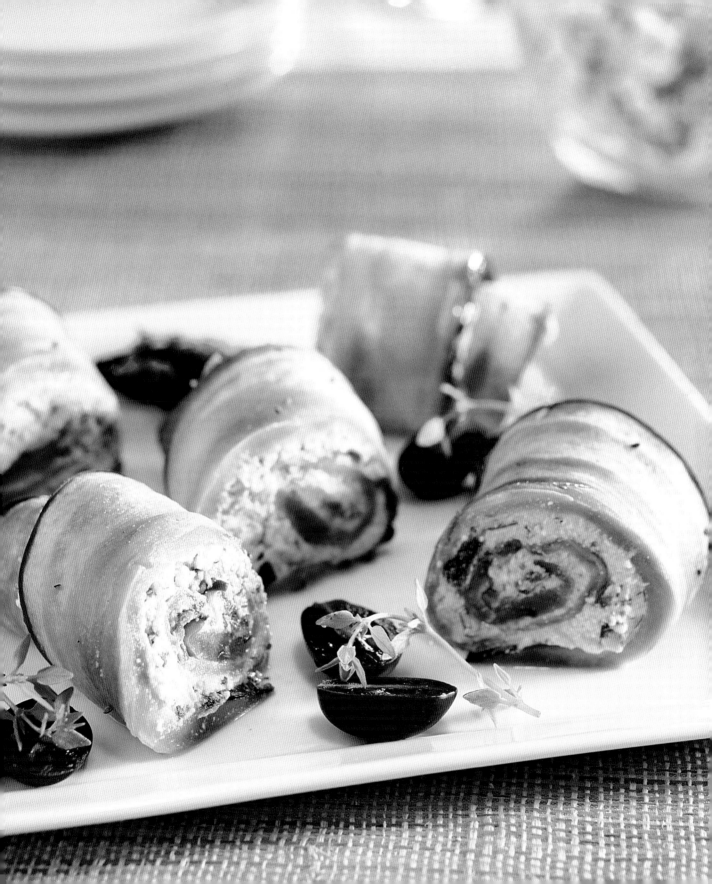

BLT CHICKEN SALAD FOR TWO

MAKES 2 SERVINGS

2 boneless skinless chicken breasts

¼ cup mayonnaise or keto salad dressing, plus additional for serving

½ teaspoon black pepper

4 large lettuce leaves

1 tomato, seeded and diced

3 slices bacon, crisp-cooked and crumbled

1 hard-cooked egg,* chopped

See deviled egg recipe on page 22 for instructions on making hard-cooked eggs.

1 Prepare grill for direct cooking.

2 Brush chicken with ¼ cup mayonnaise; sprinkle with pepper. Grill over medium heat 5 to 7 minutes per side or until no longer pink in center. Cool slightly; cut into thin strips.

3 Arrange lettuce on serving plates. Top with chicken, tomato, bacon and egg. Spoon additional mayonnaise over top, if desired.

NUTRIENTS PER SERVING (SERVING SIZE: ½ OF TOTAL RECIPE)

CALORIES 426   **TOTAL FAT** 30g   **CARBS** 5g   **NET CARBS** 4g   **DIETARY FIBER** 1g   **PROTEIN** 34g

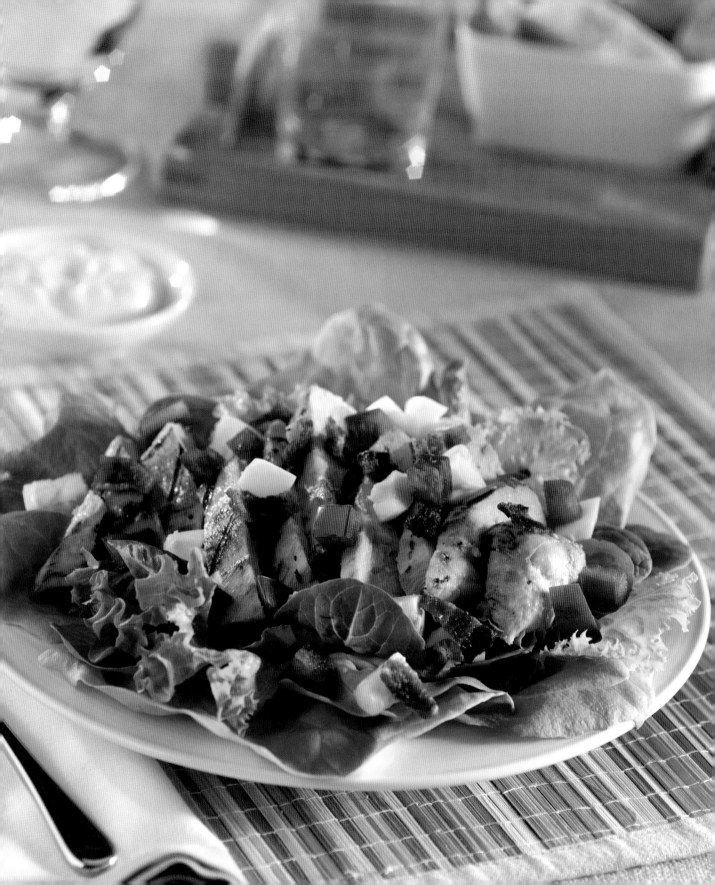

KALE WITH CARAMELIZED GARLIC

MAKES 6 SERVINGS

1½ pounds fresh kale, tough stems removed and discarded, leaves thinly sliced (16 cups)

2 cups water

1 teaspoon salt, divided

1 tablespoon olive oil

8 cloves garlic, thinly sliced

1 teaspoon red wine vinegar

⅛ to ¼ teaspoon red pepper flakes

1 Place kale, water and ½ teaspoon salt in large saucepan; bring to a boil over medium-high heat. Cover and cook 6 to 8 minutes or until kale is tender but still bright green. Drain well.

2 Meanwhile, heat oil in large nonstick skillet over medium heat. Add garlic; cook and stir 4 minutes or until garlic is golden brown, being careful not to allow garlic to burn. Add kale, vinegar, remaining ½ teaspoon salt and red pepper flakes; cook and stir until heated through.

NUTRIENTS PER SERVING (SERVING SIZE: ½ CUP)

CALORIES 80 **TOTAL FAT** 3g **CARBS** 11g **NET CARBS** 7g **DIETARY FIBER** 4g **PROTEIN** 5g

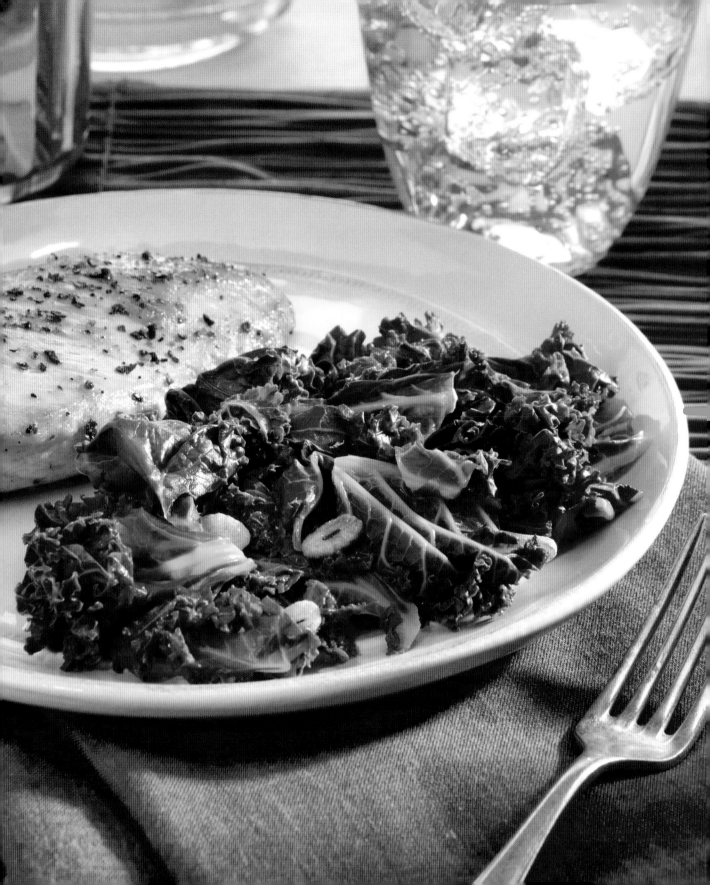

HERBED ZUCCHINI RIBBONS

MAKES 4 SERVINGS

3 small zucchini (about ¾ pound total)

2 tablespoons olive oil

1 tablespoon white wine vinegar

2 teaspoons chopped fresh basil leaves *or* ½ teaspoon dried basil

½ teaspoon red pepper flakes

¼ teaspoon ground coriander

Salt and black pepper

Finely chopped roasted red pepper or pimientos (optional)

1 Cut tip and stem ends from zucchini with paring knife. Using vegetable peeler, begin at stem end and make continuous ribbons down length of each zucchini.

2 Place steamer basket in large saucepan; add 1 inch of water. (Water should not touch bottom of basket.) Place zucchini ribbons in steamer basket. Cover and bring to a boil over high heat. When pan begins to steam, check zucchini for doneness. (It should be crisp-tender.) Transfer zucchini to serving dish with slotted spatula or tongs.

3 Whisk oil, vinegar, basil, red pepper flakes and coriander in small bowl until well blended.

4 Pour dressing over zucchini ribbons; toss gently to coat. Season with salt and black pepper. Garnish with roasted red pepper. Serve immediately or refrigerate up to 2 days.

NUTRIENTS PER SERVING (SERVING SIZE: ¼ OF TOTAL RECIPE)

CALORIES 80   **TOTAL FAT** 7g   **CARBS** 3g   **NET CARBS** 2g   **DIETARY FIBER** 1g   **PROTEIN** 1g

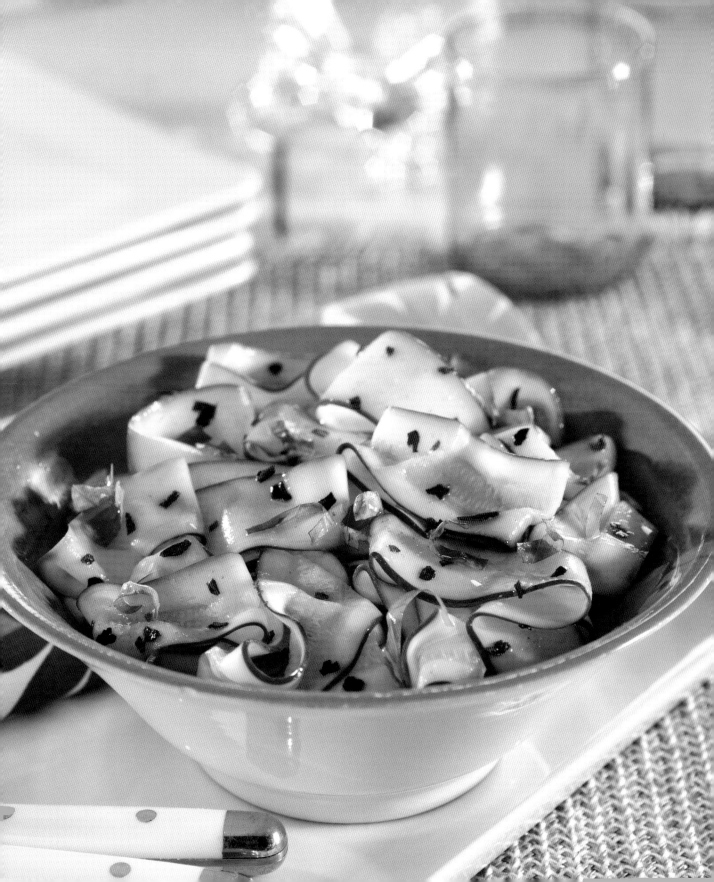

LAYERED CAPRESE SALAD

MAKES 4 SERVINGS

- 2 tablespoons extra virgin olive oil
- 2 teaspoons balsamic vinegar
- 2 cloves garlic, minced
  Salt and black pepper
- ½ small red onion, thinly sliced
- 3 medium tomatoes, sliced
- ½ cup (2 ounces) shredded mozzarella cheese
- 2 tablespoons chopped fresh parsley
- 2 tablespoons shredded fresh basil

1 Whisk oil, vinegar, garlic, salt and pepper in small bowl until well blended.

2 Spread half of onion in serving dish. Layer with half of tomatoes and sprinkle with half of cheese, parsley and basil. Drizzle with half of dressing. Repeat layers. Serve at room temperature or cover and refrigerate for 1 hour to serve chilled.

NUTRIENTS PER SERVING (SERVING SIZE: ¼ OF TOTAL RECIPE)

CALORIES 94   **TOTAL FAT** 5g   **CARBS** 9g   **NET CARBS** 6g   **DIETARY FIBER** 3g   **PROTEIN** 5g

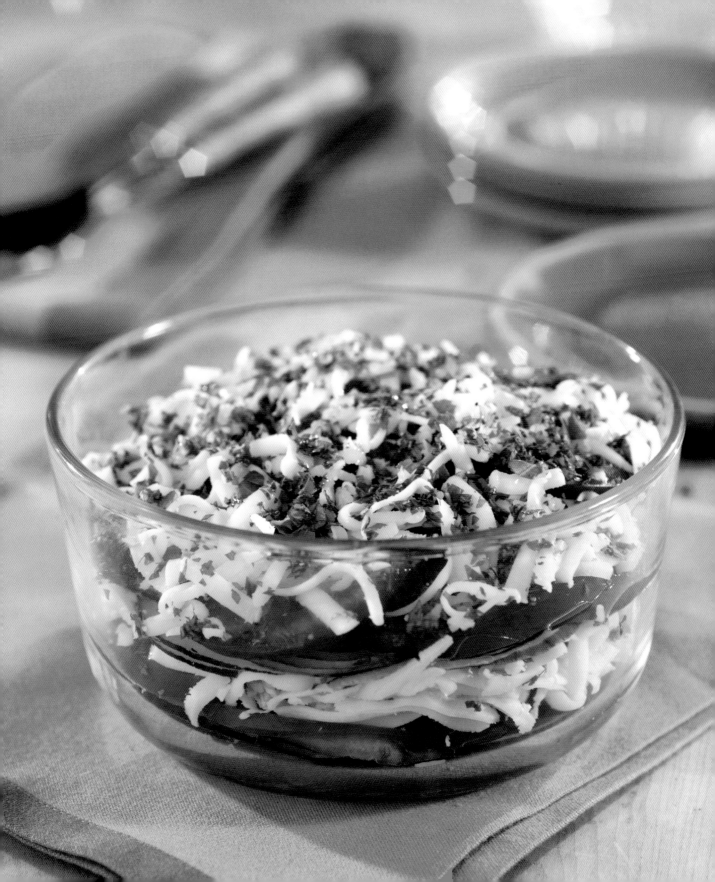

MARINATED ANTIPASTO

MAKES ABOUT 5 CUPS (10 SERVINGS)

¼ cup extra virgin olive
 oil

2 tablespoons balsamic
 vinegar

1 clove garlic, minced

½ teaspoon salt

¼ teaspoon black pepper

1 pint (2 cups) cherry
 tomatoes

1 can (about 14 ounces)
 quartered artichoke
 hearts, drained

8 ounces small balls
 or cubes fresh
 mozzarella cheese

1 cup drained pitted
 kalamata olives

¼ cup sliced fresh basil
 leaves

 Lettuce leaves

1 Whisk oil, vinegar, garlic, salt and pepper in medium bowl. Add tomatoes, artichokes, mozzarella, olives and basil; toss to coat. Let stand at room temperature 30 minutes.

2 Line platter with lettuce. Arrange antipasto over lettuce; serve at room temperature.

SERVING SUGGESTION

Antipasto makes a great snack or appetizer. Serve it in a large bowl with toothpicks or portion it into small individual serving bowls for an impressive appetizer.

NUTRIENTS PER SERVING (SERVING SIZE: ½ CUP)

CALORIES 130   **TOTAL FAT** 11g   **CARBS** 6g   **NET CARBS** 3g   **DIETARY FIBER** 3g   **PROTEIN** 5g

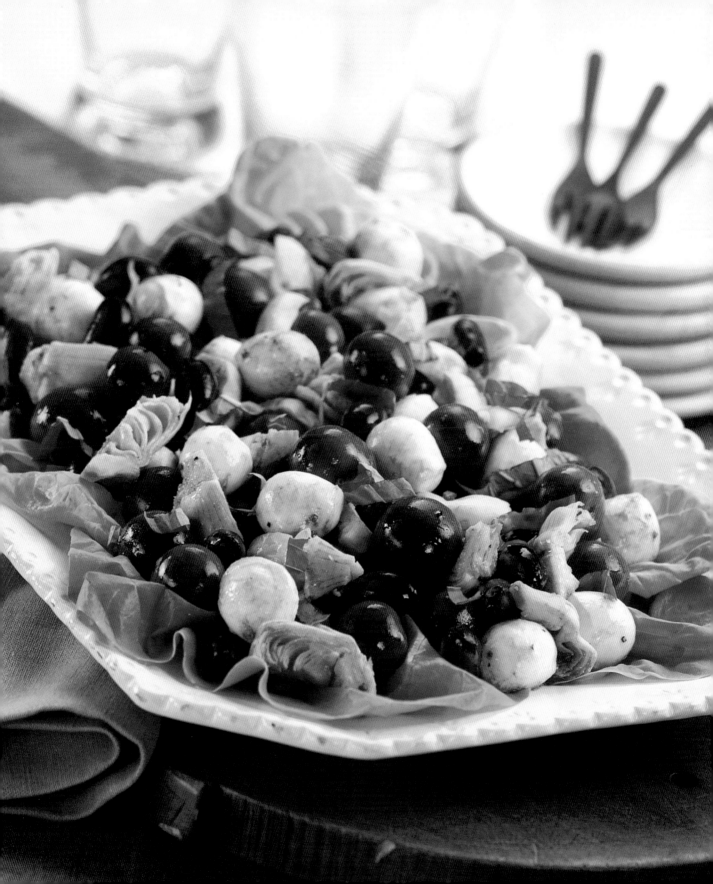

SMOKY KALE CHIFFONADE

MAKES 4 SERVINGS

¾ **pound fresh kale or mustard greens**

3 **slices bacon**

2 **tablespoons crumbled blue cheese**

1 Rinse kale well in large bowl of warm water; drain in colander. Discard any discolored leaves; trim away tough stem ends. To prepare chiffonade, stack leaves and roll up tightly from one long end. Slice crosswise into ½-inch slices; separate into strips. Set aside.

2 Cook bacon in medium skillet over medium heat until crisp. Transfer bacon to paper towels; set aside. Drain all but 1 tablespoon drippings from skillet.

3 Add kale to drippings in skillet. Cook and stir over medium-high heat 2 to 3 minutes until wilted and tender (older leaves may take slightly longer). Transfer to serving dish.

4 Crumble bacon. Add to kale with blue cheese; toss gently to blend. Serve immediately.

NUTRIENTS PER SERVING (SERVING SIZE: ¼ OF TOTAL RECIPE)

CALORIES 66　　**TOTAL FAT** 4g　　**CARBS** 5g　　**NET CARBS** 4g　　**DIETARY FIBER** 1g　　**PROTEIN** 4g

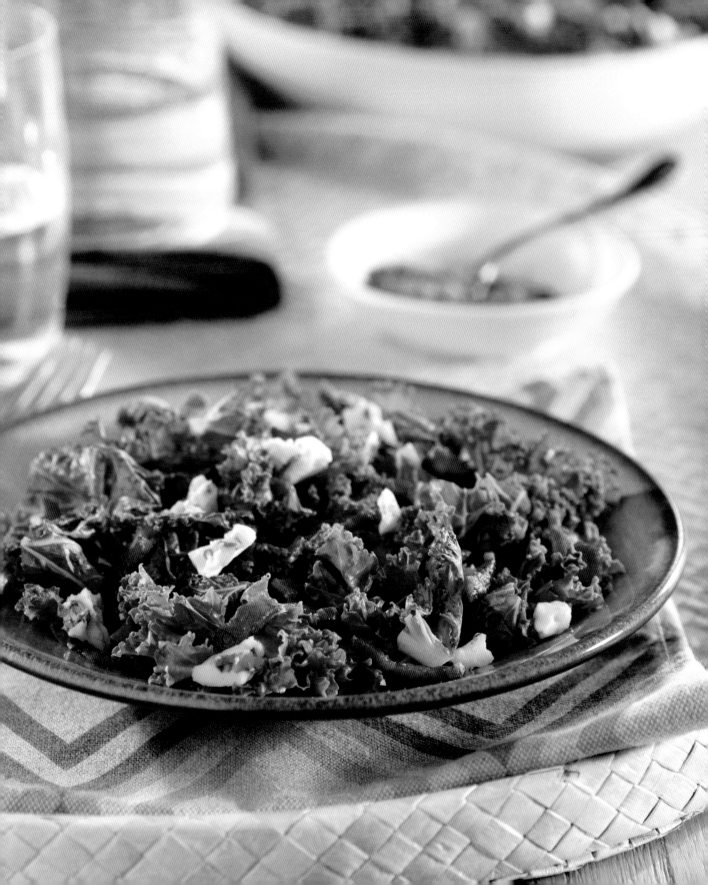

COBB SALAD

MAKES 4 SERVINGS

- 1 package (10 ounces) torn mixed salad greens *or* 8 cups torn romaine lettuce
- 6 ounces diced cooked chicken or turkey
- 1 large tomato, seeded and chopped
- ⅓ cup cooked crumbled bacon
- 1 large ripe avocado, diced

  Crumbled blue cheese

  Prepared keto blue cheese or Caesar salad dressing*

*Choose a low-carb dressing with no added sugar; do not use low-fat.

1 Place salad greens in serving bowl. Arrange chicken, tomato, bacon and avocado in rows.

2 Sprinkle with blue cheese. Serve with dressing.

SERVING SUGGESTION

This is a great way to use up leftover cooked chicken or Thanksgiving turkey.

NUTRIENTS PER SERVING (SERVING SIZE ABOUT 1 CUP OF SALAD)

CALORIES 222   **TOTAL FAT** 13g   **CARBS** 12g   **NET CARBS** 6g   **DIETARY FIBER** 6g   **PROTEIN** 17g

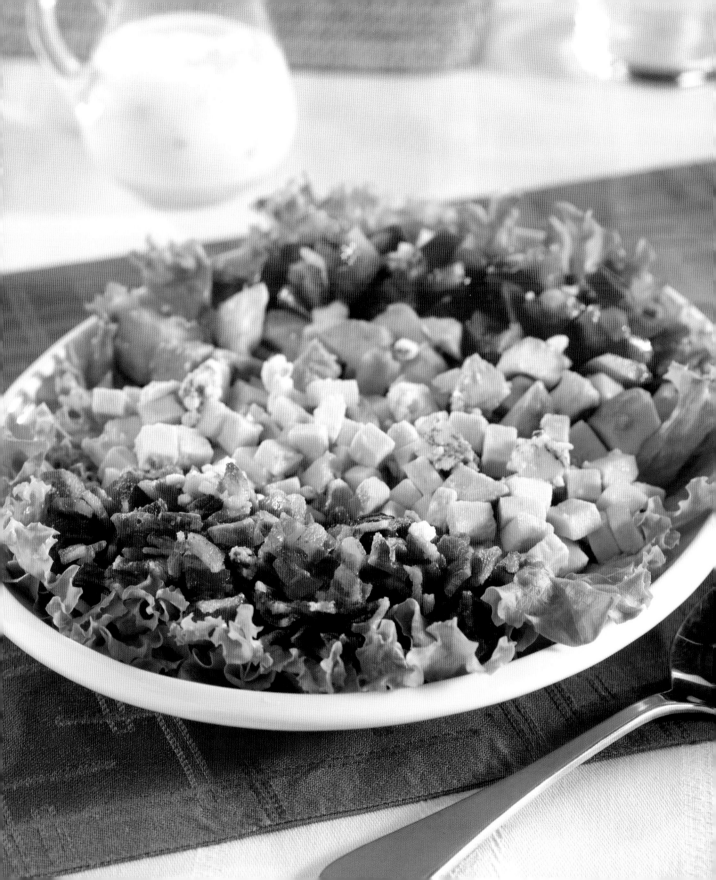

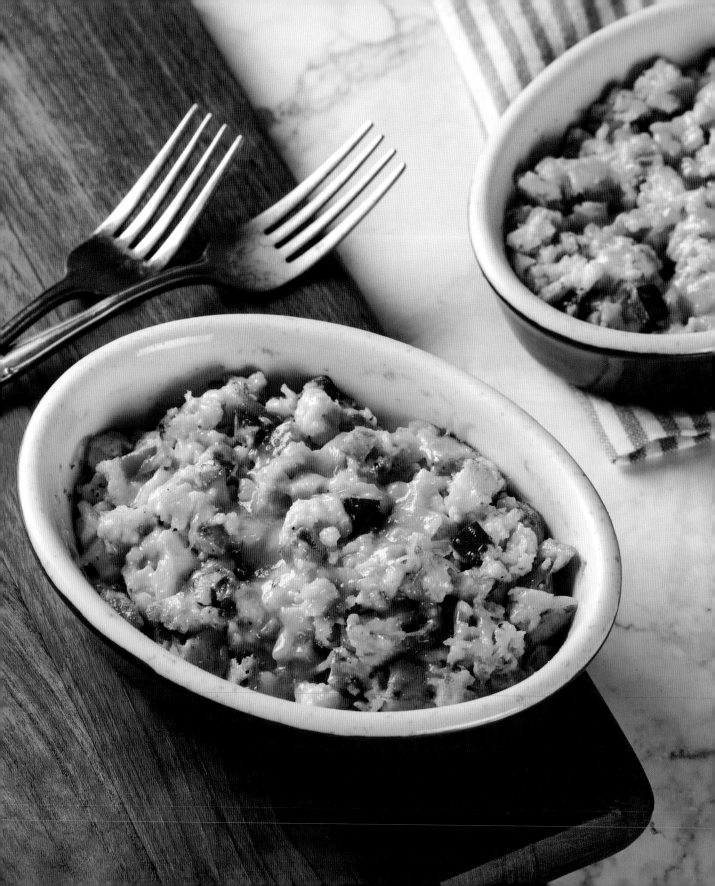

BREAKFAST AND EGG DISHES

BAKED OMELET SCRAMBLE

MAKES 2 SERVINGS

2 eggs

2 tablespoons milk

¼ teaspoon salt

⅛ teaspoon black pepper

2 tablespoons chopped red and/or green bell pepper

2 tablespoons chopped onion

¼ cup (1 ounce) shredded Cheddar cheese, divided

1 Preheat oven to 350°F. Spray one small 6×3-inch baking dish or two small ramekins with nonstick cooking spray.

2 Whisk eggs, milk, salt and black pepper in medium bowl. Add bell pepper, onion and 2 tablespoons cheese. Pour into prepared dish.

3 Bake 10 to 12 minutes or until eggs are set, stirring with fork after 5 minutes. Top with remaining cheese.

NUTRIENTS PER SERVING (SERVING SIZE: ½ OF TOTAL RECIPE)

CALORIES 110   **TOTAL FAT** 7g   **CARBS** 3g   **NET CARBS** 3g   **DIETARY FIBER** 0g   **PROTEIN** 7g

ASPARAGUS FRITTATA PROSCIUTTO CUPS

MAKES 12 CUPS

1 tablespoon olive oil

1 small red onion, finely chopped

1½ cups sliced asparagus (½-inch pieces)

1 clove garlic, minced

12 thin slices prosciutto

8 eggs

½ cup (2 ounces) grated white Cheddar cheese

¼ cup grated Parmesan cheese

2 tablespoons whipping cream

⅛ teaspoon black pepper

1 Preheat oven to 375°F. Spray 12 standard (2½-inch) muffin cups with nonstick cooking spray.

2 Heat oil in large skillet over medium heat. Add onion; cook and stir 4 minutes or until softened. Add asparagus and garlic; cook and stir 8 minutes or until asparagus is crisp-tender. Set aside to cool slightly.

3 Line each prepared muffin cup with prosciutto slice. (Prosciutto should cover cup as much as possible, with edges extending above muffin pan.) Whisk eggs, Cheddar, Parmesan, cream and pepper in large bowl until well blended. Stir in asparagus mixture. Pour into prosciutto-lined cups, filling about three-fourths full.

4 Bake about 20 minutes or until frittatas are puffed and golden brown and edges are pulling away from pan. Cool in pan 10 minutes. Remove to wire rack; serve warm or at room temperature.

NUTRIENTS PER SERVING (SERVING SIZE: 2 CUPS)

CALORIES 270   **TOTAL FAT** 18g   **CARBS** 5g   **NET CARBS** 4g   **DIETARY FIBER** 1g   **PROTEIN** 22g

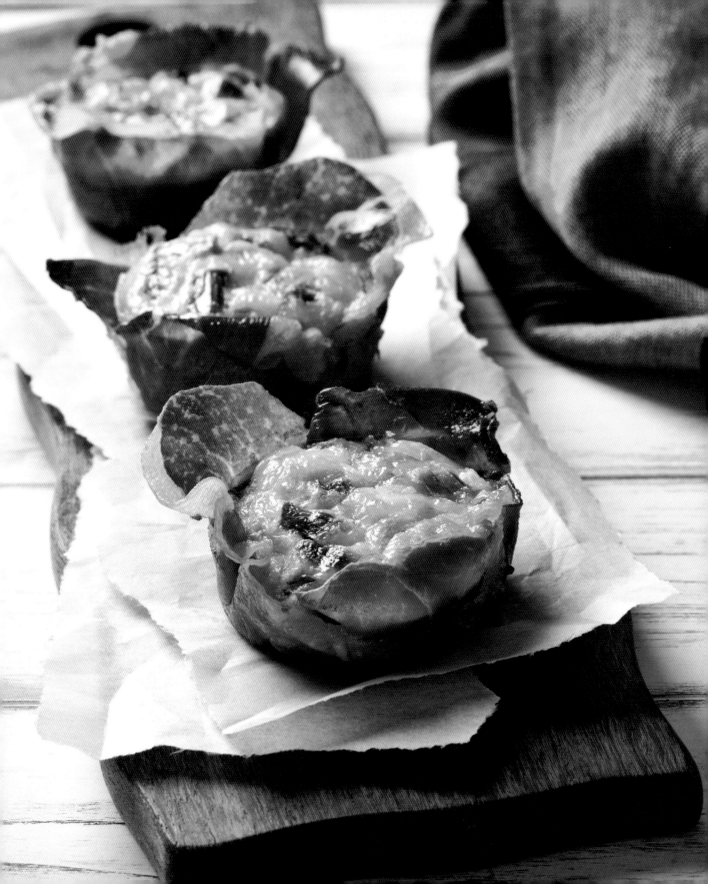

KETO EVERYTHING BAGELS
MAKES 12 BAGELS

6 eggs at room temperature,* separated

¼ teaspoon cream of tartar

2 cups almond flour

3½ teaspoons baking powder

½ teaspoon salt

¼ teaspoon garlic powder

6 tablespoons butter, melted and cooled slightly

½ cup finely shredded Asiago cheese

2 tablespoons everything bagel seasoning

To quickly warm eggs from the refrigerator, fill a bowl with warm tap water. Add the eggs and let them stand until they don't feel cold.

1 Preheat oven to 350°F. Spray 12 cavities of doughnut pans with nonstick cooking spray.

2 Place egg whites and cream of tartar in large bowl; attach whisk attachment to stand mixer. Whip egg whites on high speed 2 minutes or until stiff peaks form. Transfer egg whites to medium bowl.

3 Combine almond flour, baking powder, salt and garlic powder in mixer bowl. Add melted butter and egg yolks; mix on medium speed until well blended. Add cheese; mix well.

4 Stir one third of egg whites into almond flour mixture with spatula until well blended. Gently fold in remaining egg whites until thoroughly blended. Scoop mixture into large resealable food storage bag; cut off one corner. Pipe about ¼ cup batter into each doughnut cavity. Sprinkle each with ½ teaspoon everything bagel seasoning.

5 Bake about 10 minutes or until bagels are golden brown and set. Cool in pans 2 minutes. Remove to wire rack; serve warm or cool completely.

EVERYTHING BAGEL MUFFINS

If you don't have doughnut pans or would prefer to make muffins instead, scoop batter into 12 greased standard muffin pan cups. Sprinkle with bagel seasoning. Bake 15 minutes or until tops are golden brown and toothpick inserted into centers comes out clean.

NUTRIENTS PER SERVING (SERVING SIZE: 1 BAGEL)

CALORIES 210   **TOTAL FAT** 19g   **CARBS** 5g   **NET CARBS** 3g   **DIETARY FIBER** 2g   **PROTEIN** 8g

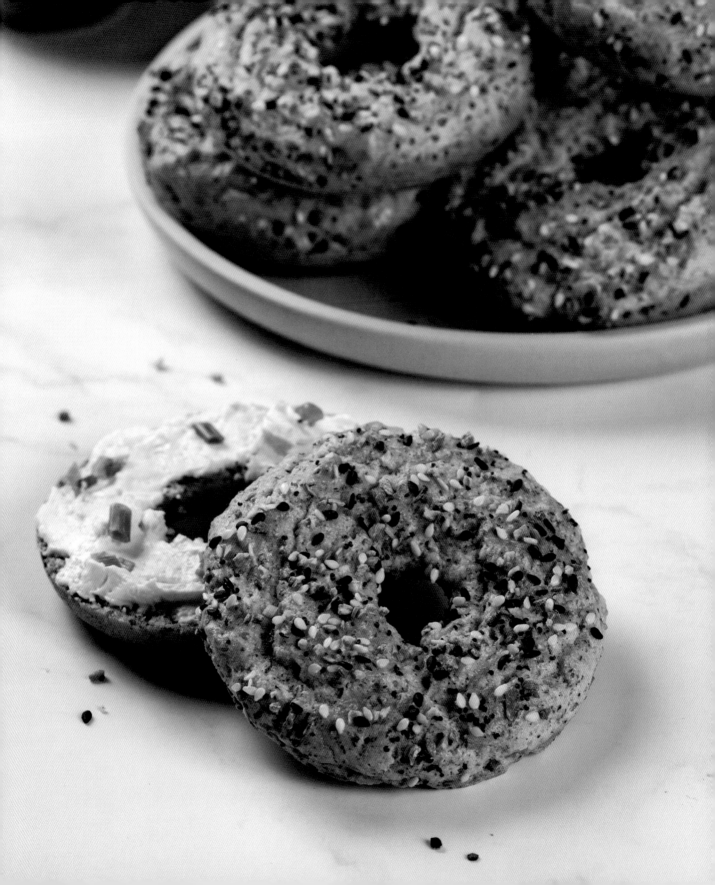

BACON AND EGG BREAKFAST CASSEROLE

MAKES 6 SERVINGS

CRUST

- 2 cups riced cauliflower (fresh or frozen)
- ½ cup shredded Parmesan cheese
- 1 egg
- ½ teaspoon salt
- ⅛ teaspoon ground red pepper (optional)

FILLING

- 1 package (about 12 ounces) bacon, chopped
- 1 onion, chopped
- 1 jalapeño pepper, seeded and chopped
- 2 cloves garlic, minced
- 1 cup (4 ounces) shredded Cheddar cheese, divided
- 8 eggs
- ¾ cup milk
- ¼ teaspoon salt

1 Preheat oven to 400°F. Place cauliflower in 8-inch glass baking dish; cover with plastic wrap and cut slit to vent. Microwave on HIGH 6 minutes. Remove cover; cool slightly. Press cauliflower with paper towels to remove excess moisture. Add Parmesan cheese, 1 egg, ½ teaspoon salt and red pepper, if desired; mix well. Press onto bottom and up side of baking dish. Bake 15 minutes. Remove from oven. *Reduce oven temperature to 350°F.*

2 Meanwhile, cook bacon in large skillet over medium heat until crisp. Remove with slotted spoon to paper towels to drain. Drain all but 1 tablespoon drippings from skillet; heat over medium heat. Add onion; cook and stir 5 minutes or until onion is softened. Add jalapeño and garlic; cook and stir 30 seconds. Remove from heat. Place onion mixture and all but ¼ cup bacon in crust; sprinkle with ¾ cup Cheddar.

3 Whisk eggs, milk and ¼ teaspoon salt in large bowl until well blended. Pour into crust.

4 Bake 30 minutes. Sprinkle with remaining ¼ cup Cheddar and remaining bacon; bake 5 minutes or until cheese is melted. Cut into six squares to serve.

NUTRIENTS PER SERVING (SERVING SIZE: 1 SQUARE)

CALORIES	TOTAL FAT	CARBS	NET CARBS	DIETARY FIBER	PROTEIN
470	36g	10g	8g	2g	27g

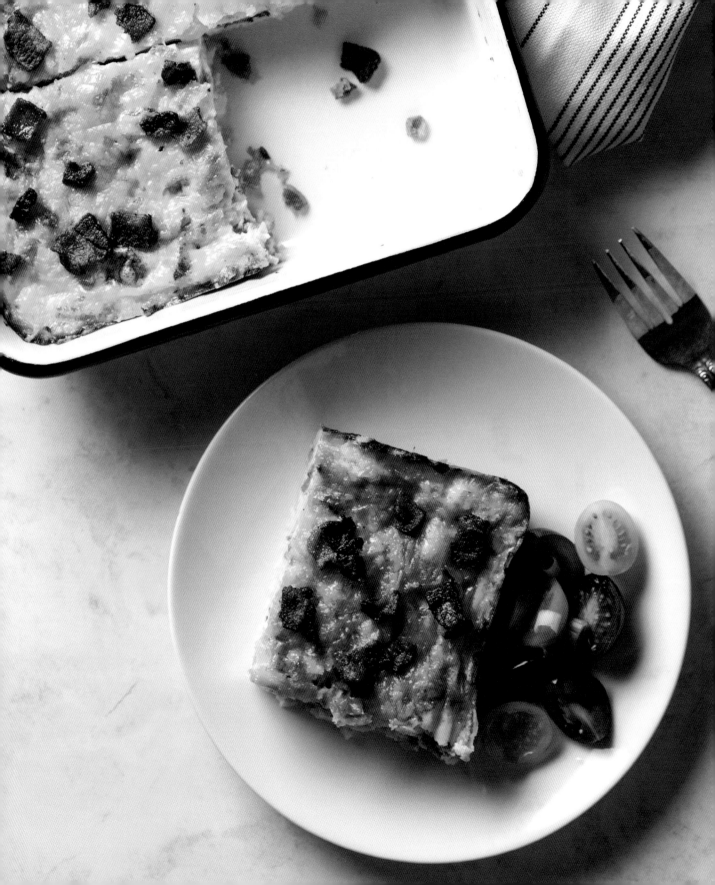

MINI SPINACH FRITTATAS
MAKES 12 MINI FRITTATAS

1 tablespoon olive oil

½ cup chopped onion

8 eggs

¼ cup plain yogurt

1 package (10 ounces) frozen chopped spinach, thawed and squeezed dry

½ cup (2 ounces) shredded white Cheddar cheese

¼ cup grated Parmesan cheese

¾ teaspoon salt

⅛ teaspoon black pepper

⅛ teaspoon ground red pepper

Dash ground nutmeg

1 Preheat oven to 350°F. Spray 12 standard (2½-inch) muffin cups with nonstick cooking spray.

2 Heat oil in large nonstick skillet over medium heat. Add onion; cook and stir about 5 minutes or until tender. Set aside to cool slightly.

3 Whisk eggs and yogurt in large bowl. Stir in spinach, Cheddar, Parmesan, salt, black pepper, red pepper, nutmeg and onion until blended. Divide mixture evenly among prepared muffin cups.

4 Bake 20 to 25 minutes or until eggs are puffed and firm and no longer shiny. Cool in pan 2 minutes. Loosen bottom and sides with small spatula or knife; remove to wire rack. Serve warm, cold or at room temperature.

NUTRIENTS PER SERVING (SERVING SIZE: 3 FRITTATAS)

CALORIES 290 **TOTAL FAT** 20g **CARBS** 6g **NET CARBS** 4g **DIETARY FIBER** 2g **PROTEIN** 21g

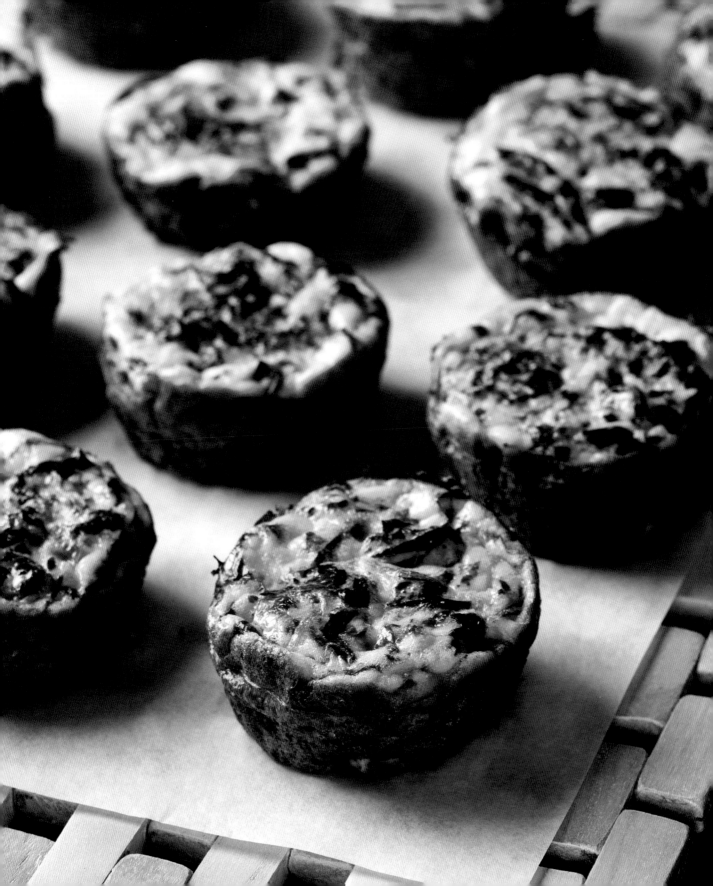

BACON-KALE QUICHE
MAKES 6 SERVINGS

CRUST

- ¾ cup coconut flour
- ¾ cup almond flour
- ¼ teaspoon salt
- 2 eggs
- 6 tablespoons coconut oil or butter, melted

FILLING

- 8 eggs
- ½ cup whipping cream
- 1 package (12 ounces) bacon
- 3 cups tightly packed chopped stemmed kale
- 1 cup chopped onion
- ½ cup finely shredded Parmesan cheese
- ¼ cup finely chopped sun-dried tomatoes

1 Preheat oven to 375°F. Combine coconut flour, almond flour and salt in medium bowl. Stir in 2 eggs and coconut oil until well blended. Press onto bottom and up side of deep dish pie plate. Bake 5 minutes.

2 Whisk eggs and cream in large bowl until well blended. Cook bacon in large skillet until crisp. Drain on paper towels; chop when cool enough to handle. Add kale and onion to drippings in skillet; cook and stir over medium heat about 5 minutes or until onion is golden and kale is wilted. Add vegetables and drippings to eggs; mix well. Stir in cheese, tomatoes and bacon. Pour into prepared crust.

3 Bake 40 minutes or until quiche is puffed and knife inserted into center comes out clean, covering edges of crust with foil after 20 minutes to prevent overbrowning. Let stand 20 minutes before cutting into six wedges.

NUTRIENTS PER SERVING (SERVING SIZE: 1 WEDGE)

CALORIES	TOTAL FAT	CARBS	NET CARBS	DIETARY FIBER	PROTEIN
730	61g	17g	9g	8g	26g

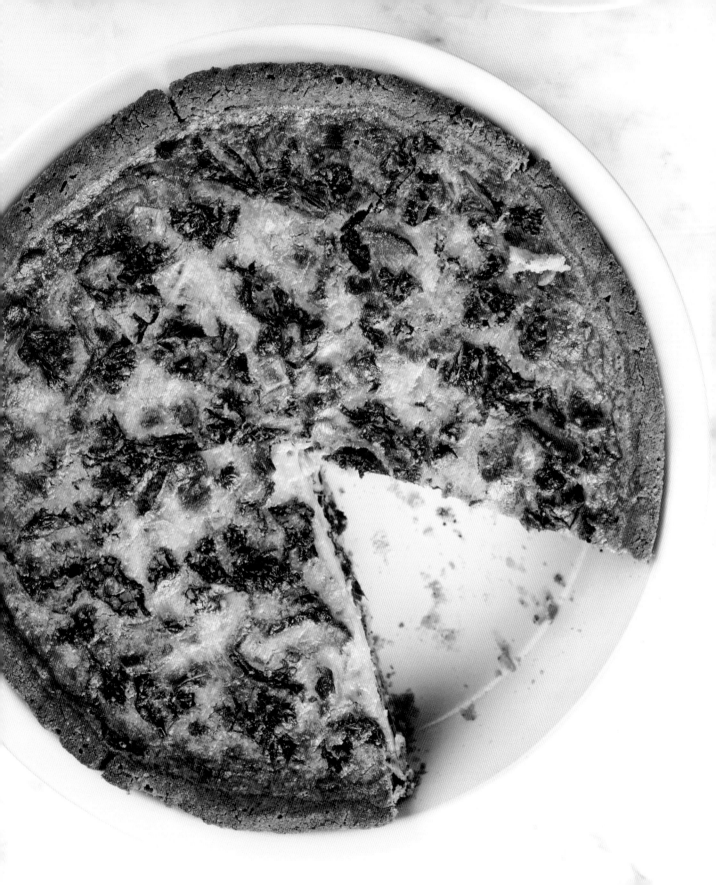

ZUCCHINI-TOMATO FRITTATA

MAKES 4 SERVINGS

½ cup sun-dried tomatoes not packed in oil (1 ounce)

1 cup sliced zucchini

1 cup broccoli florets

1 cup diced red or yellow bell pepper

3 whole eggs*

5 egg whites*

½ cup cottage cheese

¼ cup chopped green onions

¼ cup chopped fresh basil

⅛ teaspoon ground red pepper

2 tablespoons grated Parmesan cheese

Or substitute with 1½ cups liquid egg substitute or 6 whole eggs.

1 Place tomatoes in small bowl. Pour 1 cup boiling water over tomatoes; let stand 10 minutes. Drain and coarsely chop.

2 Preheat broiler. Spray 10-inch ovenproof skillet with nonstick cooking spray; heat over medium-high heat. Add zucchini, broccoli and bell pepper; cook and stir 3 to 4 minutes or until crisp-tender.

3 Whisk whole eggs, egg whites, cottage cheese, tomatoes, green onions, basil and red pepper in medium bowl until well blended. Pour egg mixture over vegetables in skillet. Cook 7 to 8 minutes or until frittata is almost firm and golden brown on bottom, gently lifting sides of frittata so uncooked egg flows underneath. Remove from heat. Sprinkle with Parmesan.

4 Broil about 5 inches from heat 3 to 5 minutes or until top is golden brown. Cut into four wedges. Serve immediately.

NUTRIENTS PER SERVING (SERVING SIZE: 1 WEDGE)

CALORIES 160   **TOTAL FAT** 5g   **CARBS** 13g   **NET CARBS** 10g   **DIETARY FIBER** 3g   **PROTEIN** 16g

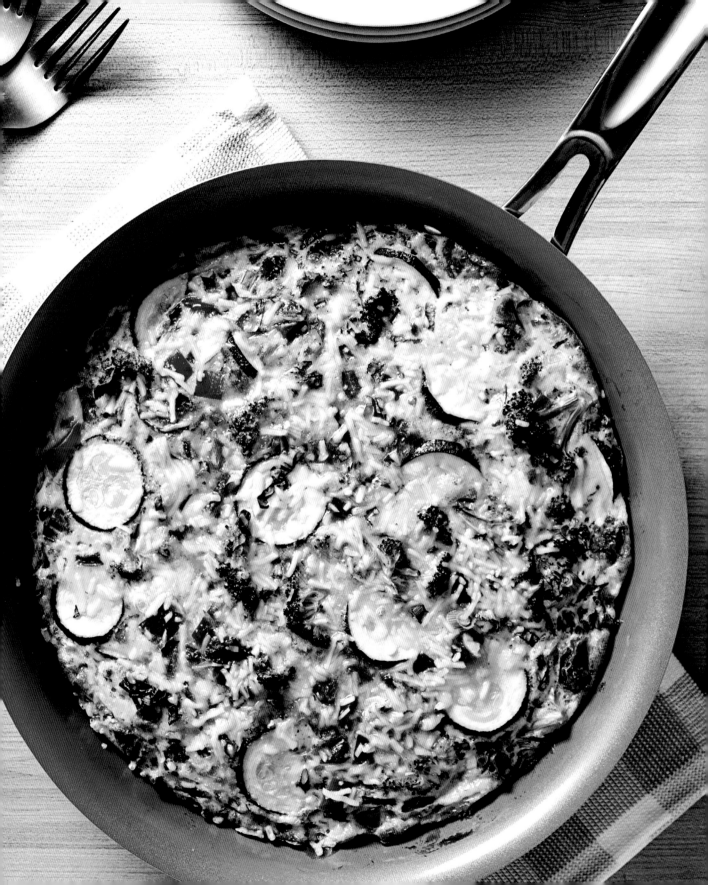

ARTICHOKE OLIVE OMELET

MAKES 2 SERVINGS

¼ cup chopped onion

¼ cup canned artichoke hearts, rinsed and drained

¼ cup chopped spinach

¼ cup chopped plum tomato

2 tablespoons sliced pitted black olives, rinsed and drained

1 cup liquid egg substitute *or* 4 eggs

Salt and black pepper

1 Spray small nonstick skillet with nonstick cooking spray; heat over medium heat. Add onion; cook and stir 2 minutes or until crisp-tender. Add artichokes; cook and stir until heated through. Add spinach, tomato and olives; stir gently. Transfer to small bowl.

2 Wipe out skillet with paper towels; spray with cooking spray. Heat skillet over medium heat. Pour egg substitute into skillet; sprinkle with salt and pepper. Cook and stir gently, lifting edge to allow uncooked portion to flow underneath. Continue cooking until set.

3 Spoon vegetable mixture over half of omelet; gently loosen omelet with spatula and fold in half. Serve immediately.

NUTRIENTS PER SERVING (SERVING SIZE: ½ OF OMELET)

CALORIES 111   **TOTAL FAT** 3g   **CARBS** 7g   **NET CARBS** 6g   **DIETARY FIBER** 1g   **PROTEIN** 13g

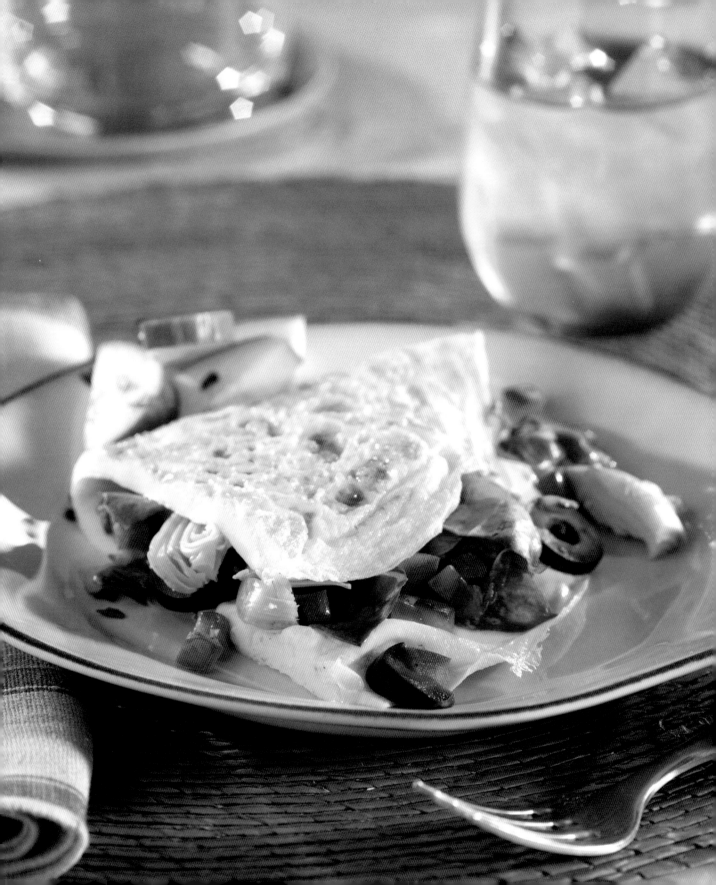

HAM AND ASPARAGUS QUICHE

MAKES 6 SERVINGS

2 cups sliced asparagus (½-inch pieces)

1 red bell pepper, chopped

1 tablespoon water

1 cup milk

4 egg whites

1 whole egg

4 ounces chopped cooked deli ham

2 tablespoons chopped fresh tarragon or basil

2 tablespoons minced green onion

1 clove garlic, minced

½ teaspoon salt

¼ teaspoon black pepper

½ cup (2 ounces) finely shredded Swiss cheese

1 Preheat oven to 350°F. Spray 9-inch pie plate with nonstick cooking spray.

2 Combine asparagus, bell pepper and water in microwavable bowl. Cover with plastic wrap; cut slit to vent. Microwave on HIGH 2 minutes or until vegetables are crisp-tender. Drain vegetables.

3 Whisk milk, egg whites and whole egg in large bowl until well blended. Stir in vegetables, ham, tarragon, green onion, garlic, salt and black pepper. Pour into prepared pie plate.

4 Bake 35 minutes. Sprinkle cheese over quiche; bake 5 minutes or until center is set and cheese is melted. Let stand 5 minutes before serving. Cut into six wedges.

NUTRIENTS PER SERVING (SERVING SIZE: 1 WEDGE)

CALORIES 120   **TOTAL FAT** 4g   **CARBS** 9g   **NET CARBS** 7g   **DIETARY FIBER** 2g   **PROTEIN** 13g

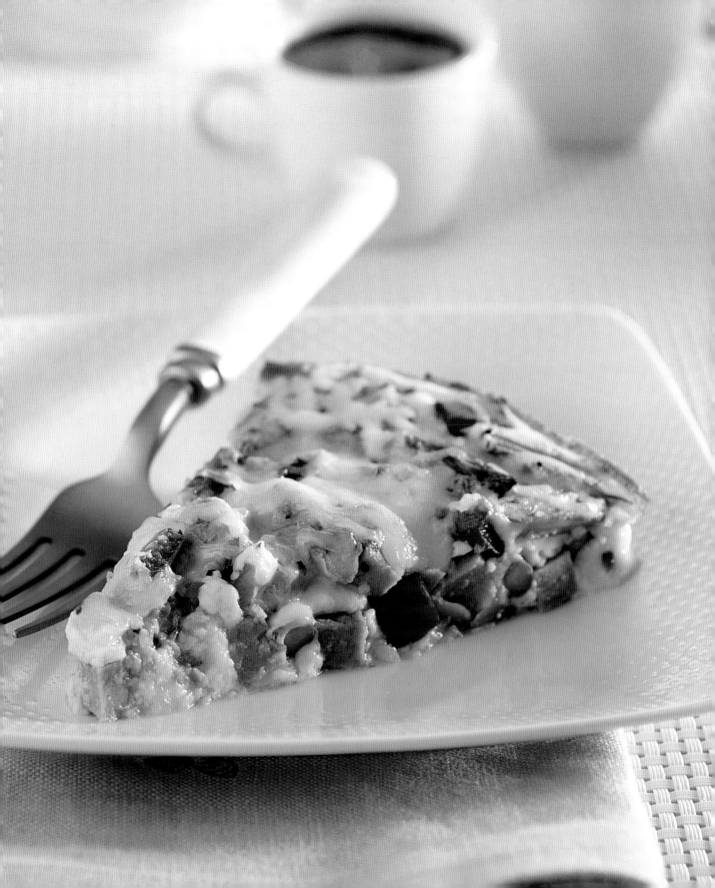

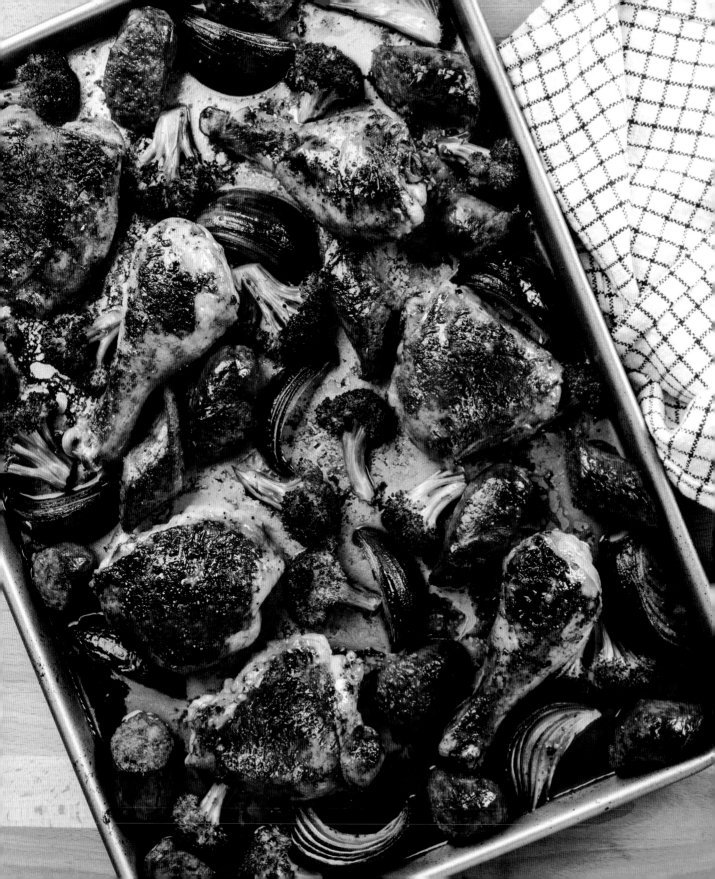

CASSEROLES
AND SHEET PAN MEALS

SHEET PAN CHICKEN AND SAUSAGE SUPPER
MAKES 6 SERVINGS

⅓ cup olive oil

2 tablespoons balsamic vinegar

1 teaspoon salt

1 teaspoon garlic powder

½ teaspoon black pepper

¼ teaspoon red pepper flakes

3 pounds bone-in skin-on chicken thighs and drumsticks

1 pound uncooked sweet Italian sausage (4 to 5 links), cut diagonally into 2-inch pieces

6 small red onions (about 1 pound), each cut into 6 wedges

3½ cups broccoli florets

1 Preheat oven to 425°F. Line sheet pan with foil, if desired, or spray with nonstick cooking spray.

2 Whisk oil, vinegar, salt, garlic powder, black pepper and red pepper flakes in small bowl until well blended. Combine chicken, sausage and onions on prepared sheet pan. Drizzle with oil mixture; toss until well coated. Spread meat and onions in single layer; turn skin side up.

3 Bake 30 minutes. Add broccoli to sheet pan; stir to coat broccoli with pan juices and turn sausage. Bake 30 minutes or until broccoli is beginning to brown and chicken is cooked through (165°F).

NUTRIENTS PER SERVING (SERVING SIZE: ⅙ OF TOTAL RECIPE)

CALORIES 430   **TOTAL FAT** 25g   **CARBS** 12g   **NET CARBS** 10g   **DIETARY FIBER** 2g   **PROTEIN** 41g

MOUSSAKA
MAKES 4 SERVINGS

1 eggplant (about 1 pound), cut into ¼-inch slices

2 tablespoons olive oil

1 pound ground beef

1 can (about 14 ounces) diced tomatoes, drained

¼ cup red wine

2 tablespoons tomato paste

¾ teaspoon salt

½ teaspoon dried oregano

¼ teaspoon ground cinnamon, plus additional for garnish

¼ teaspoon black pepper

⅛ teaspoon ground allspice

4 ounces cream cheese, softened

¼ cup milk

¼ cup grated Parmesan cheese

1 Preheat broiler. Lightly coat 8-inch square baking dish with nonstick cooking spray.

2 Line baking sheet with foil. Arrange eggplant slices on foil, overlapping slightly if necessary. Brush with oil; broil 5 to 6 inches from heat 4 minutes on each side. *Reduce oven temperature to 350°F.*

3 Meanwhile, brown beef in large nonstick skillet over medium-high heat 6 to 8 minutes, stirring to break up meat. Drain fat. Add tomatoes, wine, tomato paste, salt, oregano, ¼ teaspoon cinnamon, pepper and allspice. Bring to a boil, breaking up large pieces of tomato with spoon. Reduce heat to medium-low; cover and simmer 10 minutes.

4 Place cream cheese and milk in small microwavable bowl. Cover and microwave on HIGH 1 minute. Stir with fork until smooth.

5 Arrange half of eggplant slices in prepared baking dish. Spoon half of meat sauce over eggplant; sprinkle with half of Parmesan cheese. Repeat layers. Spoon cream cheese mixture evenly over top. Bake 20 minutes or until top begins to crack slightly. Sprinkle lightly with additional cinnamon, if desired. Let stand 10 minutes before serving.

NUTRIENTS PER SERVING (SERVING SIZE: ¼ OF TOTAL RECIPE)

CALORIES 460   **TOTAL FAT** 29g   **CARBS** 18g   **NET CARBS** 13g   **DIETARY FIBER** 5g   **PROTEIN** 30g

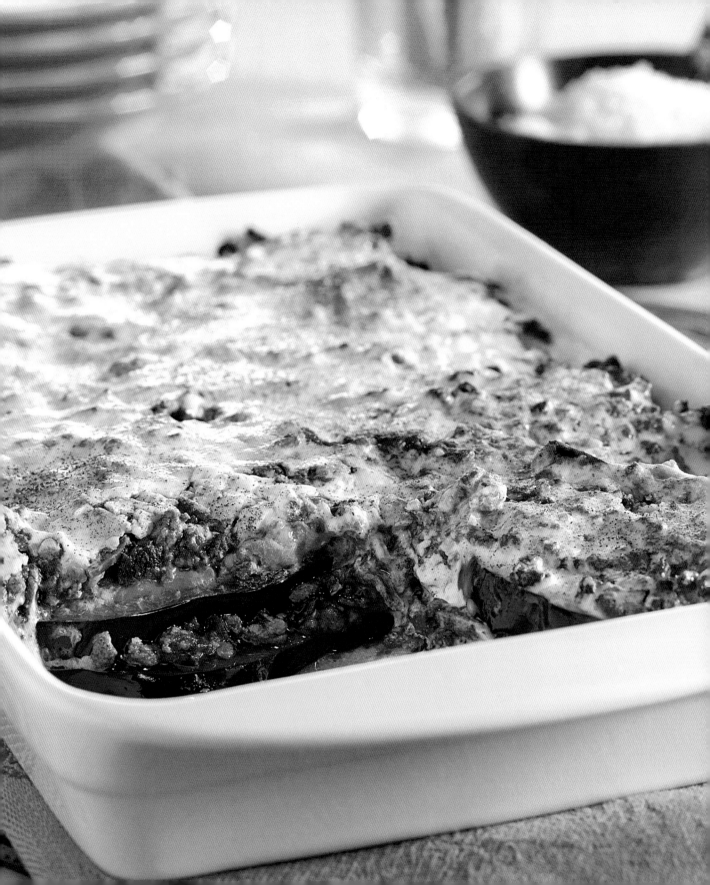

ROASTED CHICKEN WITH CABBAGE

MAKES 4 SERVINGS

⅓ cup olive oil, plus additional for pan

2 tablespoons red wine vinegar

2 cloves garlic, minced

1 teaspoon salt

1 teaspoon onion powder

¼ teaspoon paprika

¼ teaspoon black pepper

8 bone-in skin-on chicken thighs (about 3 pounds)

1½ medium onions, cut into ½-inch slices (do not separate into rings)

1 small head green cabbage (about 1½ pounds)

Chopped fresh parsley (optional)

1 Preheat oven to 425°F. Brush sheet pan with oil.

2 Whisk ⅓ cup oil, vinegar, garlic, salt, onion powder, paprika and pepper in large bowl until well blended. Remove half of mixture to medium bowl; add chicken and turn to coat.

3 Add onion slices to bowl with oil mixture; turn to coat. Arrange in single layer on prepared sheet pan. Cut cabbage in half through core (do not remove core). Cut each half into 1-inch wedges. Add cabbage to bowl with oil mixture; turn to coat. Arrange cabbage over onions on sheet pan. Place chicken, skin side up, on top of cabbage.

4 Roast 50 to 55 minutes or until chicken is 165°F. Remove chicken to plate; tent with foil to keep warm. Carefully drain liquid from sheet pan. Stir vegetables; roast 10 to 15 minutes or until edges begin to brown and cabbage is crisp-tender. Serve chicken with vegetables. Garnish with parsley.

NUTRIENTS PER SERVING (SERVING SIZE: ¼ OF TOTAL RECIPE)

CALORIES 480   **TOTAL FAT** 27g   **CARBS** 15g   **NET CARBS** 10g   **DIETARY FIBER** 5g   **PROTEIN** 43g

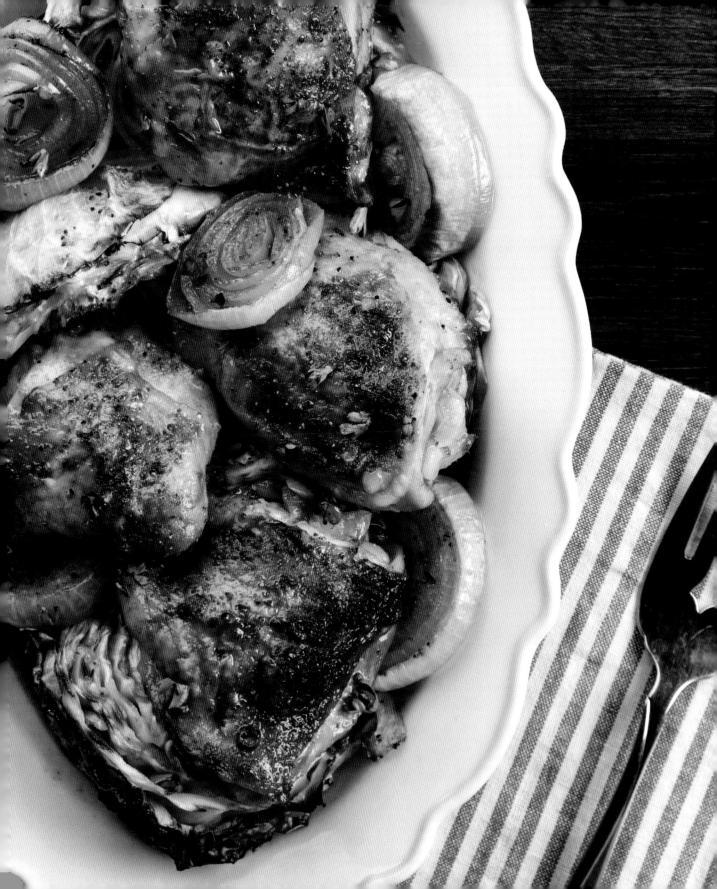

CAULIFLOWER, SAUSAGE AND GOUDA SHEET PAN

MAKES 6 SERVINGS

1 package (16 ounces) white mushrooms, stemmed and halved

3 tablespoons olive oil, divided

1 teaspoon salt, divided

1 head cauliflower, separated into florets and thinly sliced

¼ teaspoon chipotle chili powder

1 package (about 13 ounces) smoked sausage, cut into ¼-inch slices

2 tablespoons Dijon mustard

½ red onion, thinly sliced

6 ounces Gouda cheese, cubed

1 Preheat oven to 400°F.

2 Place mushrooms in medium bowl. Drizzle with 1 tablespoon oil and sprinkle with ½ teaspoon salt; toss to coat. Spread on sheet pan.

3 Place cauliflower, remaining 2 tablespoons oil, ½ teaspoon salt and chipotle chili powder in same bowl; toss to coat. Spread on sheet pan with mushrooms.

4 Combine sausage and mustard in same bowl; stir until well coated. Arrange sausage over vegetables; top with onion.

5 Roast 30 minutes. Remove from oven; place cheese cubes on top of cauliflower. Bake 5 minutes or until cheese is melted and cauliflower is tender.

NUTRIENTS PER SERVING (SERVING SIZE: ⅙ OF TOTAL RECIPE)

CALORIES 340   **TOTAL FAT** 24g   **CARBS** 9g   **NET CARBS** 7g   **DIETARY FIBER** 2g   **PROTEIN** 20g

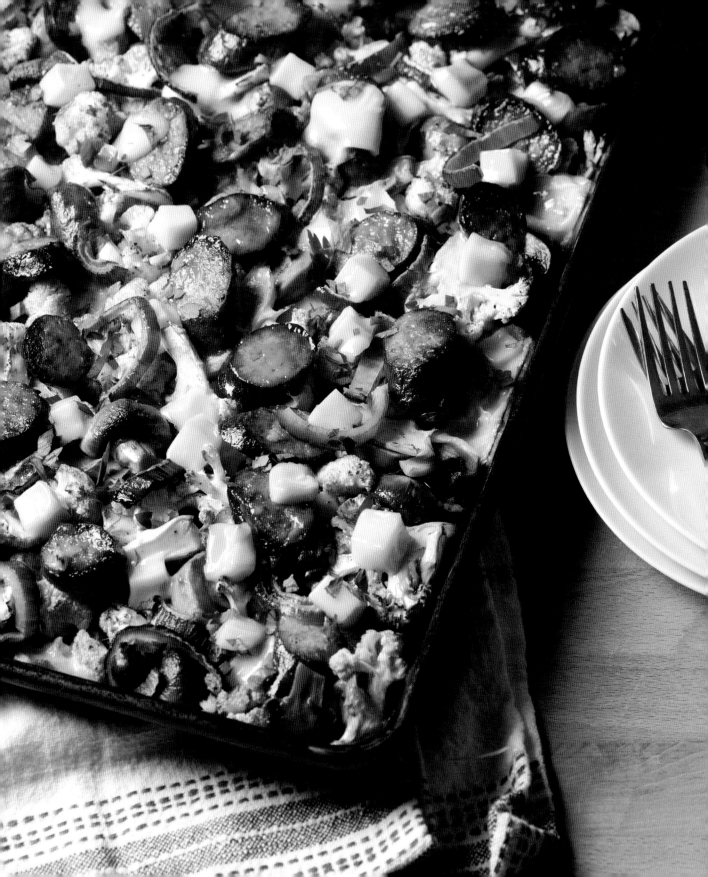

PORK TENDERLOIN WITH AVOCADO-TOMATILLO SALSA

MAKES 4 SERVINGS

1½ teaspoons chili powder
½ teaspoon salt
½ teaspoon ground cumin
1 pound pork tenderloin
1 teaspoon olive oil

SALSA

2 medium tomatillos, husked* and diced
½ ripe medium avocado, diced
1 jalapeño pepper, seeded and finely chopped
2 tablespoons finely chopped red onion
1 clove garlic, minced
1 tablespoon lime juice
1 to 2 tablespoons chopped fresh cilantro
⅛ teaspoon salt
4 lime wedges (optional)

Remove the husk by pulling from the bottom to where it attaches at the stem. Wash before using.

1 Preheat oven to 425°F. Line sheet pan with foil. Combine chili powder, ½ teaspoon salt and cumin in small bowl. Sprinkle evenly all over pork, pressing to adhere spices.

2 Heat oil in large nonstick skillet over medium-high heat. Add pork; cook 3 minutes. Turn and cook 2 to 3 minutes longer or until well browned. Place on prepared sheet pan.

3 Bake 20 to 25 minutes or until barely pink in center (about 145°F). Remove from oven and let stand 5 minutes before slicing.

4 For salsa, combine tomatillos, avocado, jalapeño, onion, garlic, lime juice, cilantro and ⅛ teaspoon salt in medium bowl; toss gently to blend. Serve with pork slices and additional lime wedges, if desired.

TIP

Choose firm tomatillos with dry husks that are not too ragged. Store in a paper bag in refrigerator for up to 1 month.

NUTRIENTS PER SERVING (SERVING SIZE: 3 OUNCES PORK AND ¼ CUP SALSA)

CALORIES 174   **TOTAL FAT** 6g   **CARBS** 4g   **NET CARBS** 2g   **DIETARY FIBER** 2g   **PROTEIN** 25g

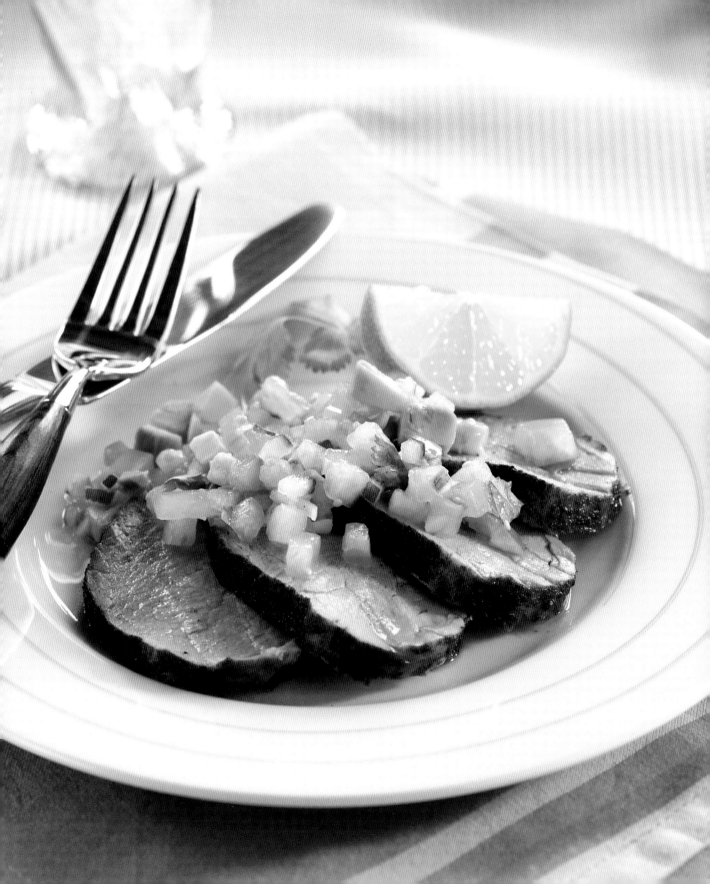

ZUCCHINI WITH FETA CASSEROLE

MAKES 4 SERVINGS

4 medium zucchini

1 tablespoon butter

2 eggs, beaten

½ cup grated Parmesan cheese

⅓ cup crumbled feta cheese

2 tablespoons chopped fresh parsley

2 teaspoons chopped fresh marjoram

Dash hot pepper sauce

Salt and black pepper

1 Preheat oven to 375°F. Spray 2-quart casserole with nonstick cooking spray.

2 Grate zucchini on large holes of box grater; drain in colander, squeezing out excess moisture. Melt butter in large skillet over medium heat. Add zucchini; cook and stir until slightly browned.

3 Remove from heat; stir in eggs, cheeses, parsley, marjoram, hot pepper sauce, salt and black pepper until well blended. Pour into prepared casserole.

4 Bake 35 minutes or until hot and bubbly.

NUTRIENTS PER SERVING (SERVING SIZE: ¼ OF TOTAL RECIPE)

CALORIES 220   **TOTAL FAT** 14g   **CARBS** 12g   **NET CARBS** 9g   **DIETARY FIBER** 3g   **PROTEIN** 15g

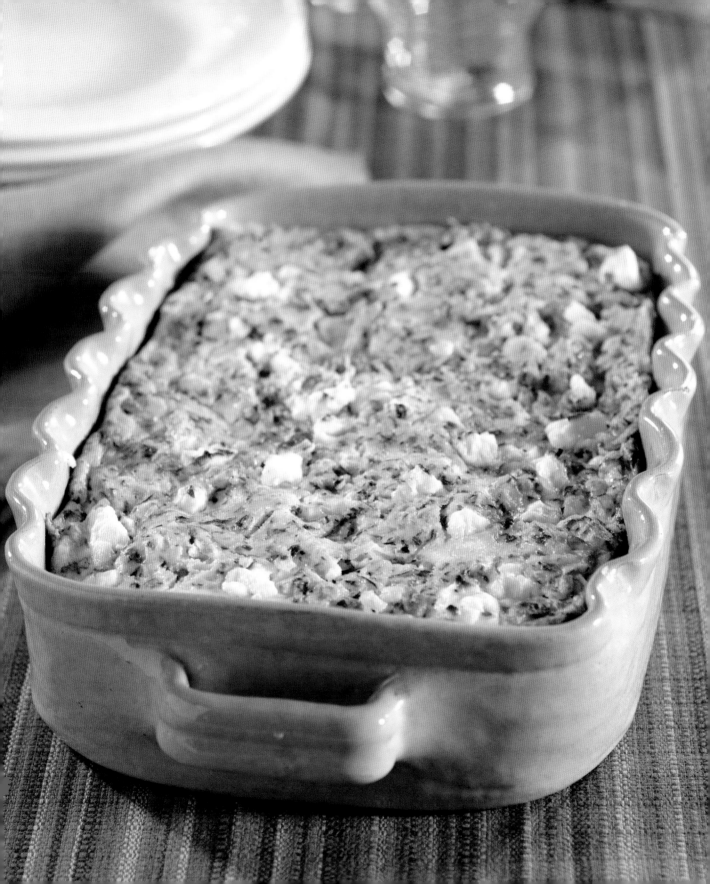

LOW-CARB LASAGNA

MAKES 15 SERVINGS

2 medium eggplants
(about 1½ pounds
total)
Salt and black pepper
1½ pounds ground beef
1½ cups marinara sauce*
1 teaspoon Italian
seasoning
½ teaspoon garlic
powder
½ teaspoon black pepper
4 cups (2 pounds) whole
milk ricotta cheese
1 egg
3 tablespoons chopped
fresh parsley,
divided
2 cups (8 ounces)
shredded mozzarella
cheese
¼ cup grated Parmesan
cheese

*Look for sauce with no
added sugar.*

1 Preheat oven to 350°F. Spray 13×9-inch baking pan
with nonstick cooking spray. Trim ends from eggplants.
Cut lengthwise into ⅛-inch-thick pieces. Place in large
colander; sprinkle with 1 tablespoon salt. Drain at least
20 minutes.

2 Meanwhile, brown ground beef in large skillet over
medium-high heat 6 to 8 minutes, stirring to break up
meat. Drain fat. Add marinara sauce, Italian seasoning,
1 teaspoon salt, garlic powder and ¼ teaspoon pepper;
cook and stir 5 minutes.

3 Combine ricotta, egg and 2 tablespoons parsley in large
bowl; stir until well blended. Season with salt and pepper.

4 Rinse eggplant slices and pat dry with paper towels.
Arrange single layer of eggplant slices in prepared
pan. Layer with half of ricotta mixture, half of sauce,
1 cup mozzarella and 2 tablespoons Parmesan. Arrange
eggplant slices over top; layer with remaining half of
ricotta mixture and half of sauce. Top with remaining
eggplant slices, remaining 1 cup mozzarella and
2 tablespoons Parmesan. Sprinkle with remaining
1 tablespoon parsley.

5 Bake uncovered 30 minutes. Tent loosely with foil and
bake additional 10 minutes or until lasagna is heated
through and sauce is bubbly.

NUTRIENTS PER SERVING (SERVING SIZE ¹⁄₁₅ OF TOTAL RECIPE)

CALORIES 314   **TOTAL FAT** 21g   **CARBS** 9g   **NET CARBS** 5g   **DIETARY FIBER** 4g   **PROTEIN** 21g

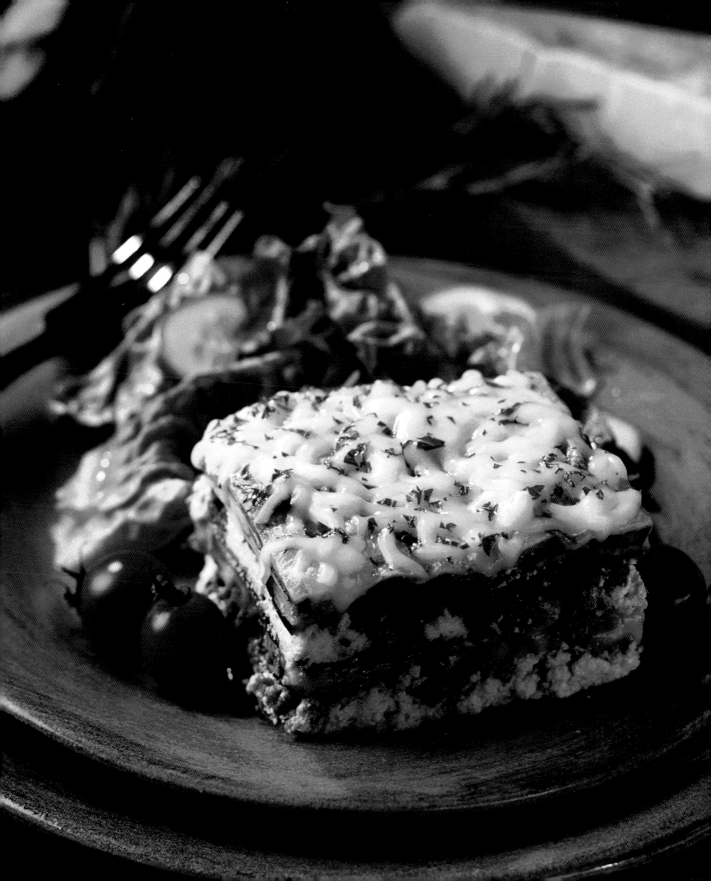

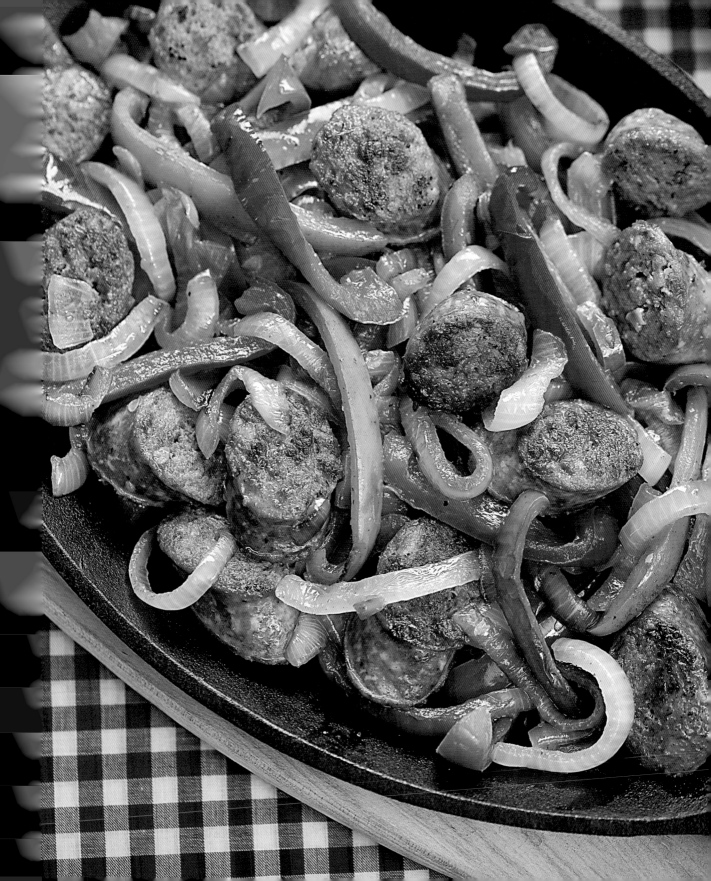

MEATY MAINS

SAUSAGE AND PEPPERS
MAKES 4 SERVINGS

- 1 pound uncooked hot or mild Italian sausage links
- 2 tablespoons olive oil
- 3 medium onions, cut into ½-inch slices
- 2 red bell peppers, cut into ½-inch slices
- 2 green bell peppers, cut into ½-inch slices
- 1½ teaspoons coarse salt, divided
- 1 teaspoon dried oregano

1 Fill medium saucepan half full with water or beer; bring to a boil over high heat. Add sausage; reduce heat to medium and cook 5 minutes. Drain and cut diagonally into 1-inch slices.

2 Heat oil in large (12-inch) cast iron skillet over medium-high heat. Add sausage; cook about 10 minutes or until browned, stirring occasionally. Transfer sausage to plate.

3 Add onions, bell peppers, 1 teaspoon salt and oregano to skillet; cook over medium heat about 10 minutes or until vegetables are very soft and browned in spots, stirring occasionally.

4 Stir sausage and remaining ½ teaspoon salt into skillet; cook 3 minutes or until heated through.

NUTRIENTS PER SERVING (SERVING SIZE: ¼ OF TOTAL RECIPE)

CALORIES 510   **TOTAL FAT** 43g   **CARBS** 15g   **NET CARBS** 11g   **DIETARY FIBER** 4g   **PROTEIN** 18g

PORK TENDERLOIN WITH CABBAGE AND LEEKS

MAKES 4 SERVINGS

- ¼ cup olive oil, plus additional for pan
- 1 teaspoon salt
- ¾ teaspoon garlic powder
- ½ teaspoon dried thyme
- ½ teaspoon black pepper
- 1 pork tenderloin (about 1¼ pounds)
- ½ medium savoy cabbage, cored and cut into ¼-inch slices (about 6 cups)
- 1 small leek, cut in half lengthwise then cut crosswise into ¼-inch diagonal slices
- 1 to 2 teaspoons cider vinegar

1 Preheat oven to 450°F. Brush baking sheet with oil.

2 Combine salt, garlic powder, thyme and pepper in small bowl; mix well. Stir in ¼ cup oil until well blended. Brush pork with about 1 tablespoon oil mixture, turning to coat all sides.

3 Combine cabbage and leek in large bowl. Drizzle with remaining oil mixture; toss to coat. Spread on prepared baking sheet; top with pork.

4 Roast about 25 minutes or until pork is 145°F, stirring cabbage mixture halfway through cooking time. Remove pork to cutting board; tent with foil and let stand 10 minutes before slicing. Add vinegar to cabbage mixture; stir to blend.

TIP

If you can't find savoy cabbage, you can substitute regular green cabbage but it may take slightly longer to cook. If the cabbage is not crisp-tender when the pork is done, return the vegetables to the oven for 10 minutes or until crisp-tender.

NUTRIENTS PER SERVING (SERVING SIZE: ¼ OF TOTAL RECIPE)

CALORIES	TOTAL FAT	CARBS	NET CARBS	DIETARY FIBER	PROTEIN
320	17g	10g	6g	4g	32g

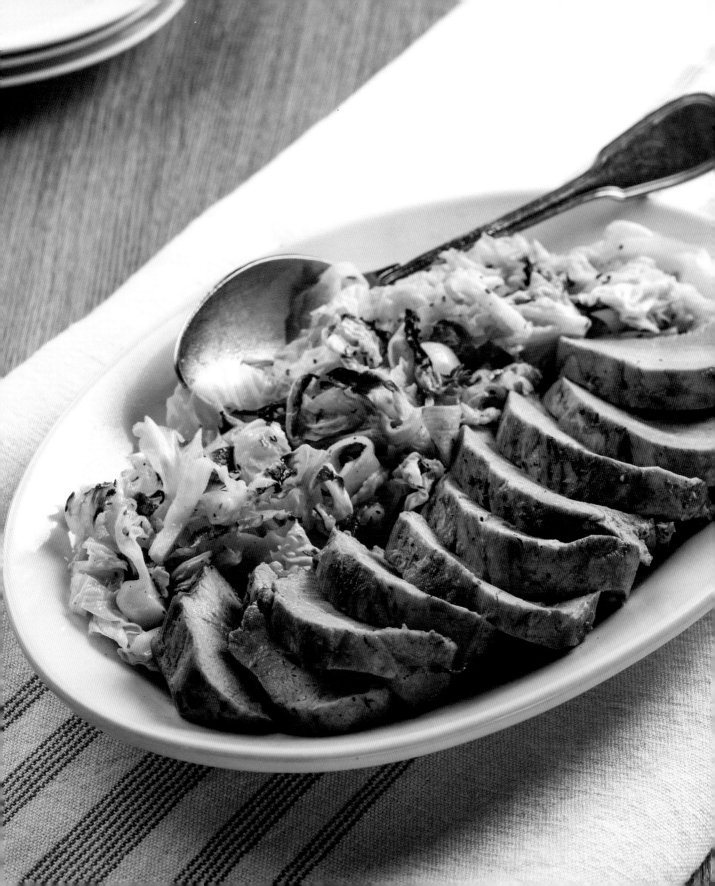

STEAK FAJITAS

MAKES 4 SERVINGS

¼ cup lime juice

¼ cup soy sauce

4 tablespoons mild olive oil, divided

2 tablespoons Worcestershire sauce

2 cloves garlic, minced

½ teaspoon ground red pepper

1 pound flank steak, skirt steak or top sirloin

1 medium yellow onion, halved and cut into ¼-inch slices

1 green bell pepper, cut into ¼-inch strips

1 red bell pepper, cut into ¼-inch strips

Lime wedges (optional)

Optional toppings: pico de gallo, guacamole, sour cream, shredded lettuce and shredded Cheddar-Jack cheese (optional)

1 Combine lime juice, soy sauce, 2 tablespoons oil, Worcestershire sauce, garlic and ground red pepper in medium bowl; mix well. Remove ¼ cup marinade to large bowl. Place steak in large resealable food storage bag. Pour remaining marinade over steak; seal bag and turn to coat. Marinate in refrigerator at least 2 hours or overnight. Add onion and bell peppers to bowl with ¼ cup marinade; toss to coat. Cover and refrigerate until ready to use.

2 Remove steak from marinade; discard marinade and wipe off excess from steak. Heat 1 tablespoon oil in large skillet (preferably cast iron) over medium-high heat. Cook steak about 4 minutes per side for medium rare or to desired doneness. Remove to cutting board; tent with foil and let rest 10 minutes.

3 Meanwhile, heat remaining 1 tablespoon oil in same skillet over medium-high heat. Drain vegetables and add to skillet; cook about 8 minutes or until vegetables are crisp-tender and beginning to brown in spots, stirring occasionally. (Cook in two batches if necessary; do not pile vegetables in skillet.)

4 Cut steak into thin slices across the grain. Serve with vegetables, lime wedges and desired toppings.

NUTRIENTS PER SERVING (SERVING SIZE: ¼ OF TOTAL RECIPE)

CALORIES 310 **TOTAL FAT** 20g **CARBS** 7g **NET CARBS** 6g **DIETARY FIBER** 1g **PROTEIN** 26g

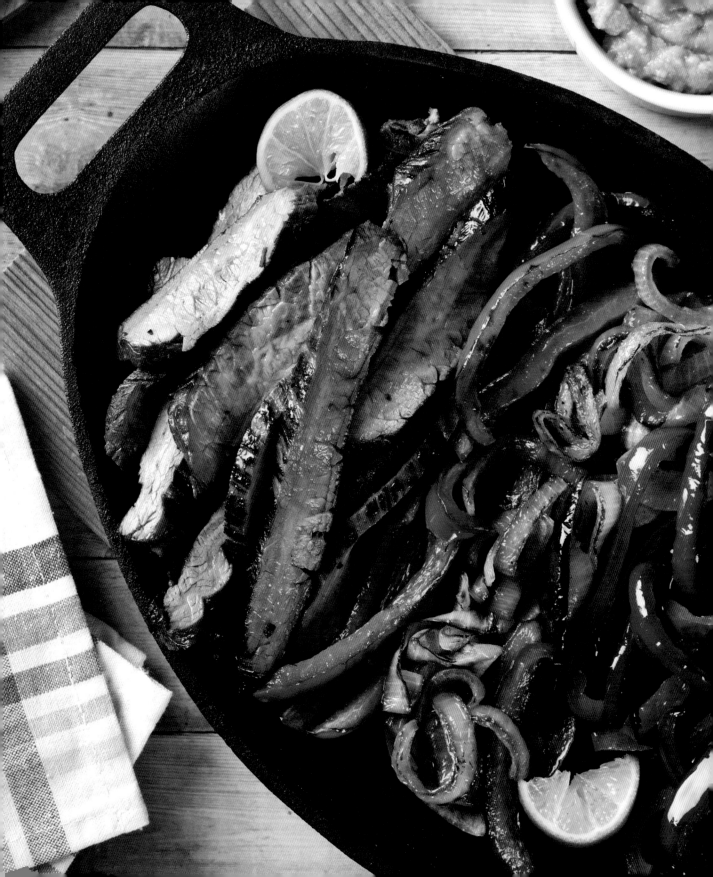

ROSEMARY PORK WITH GARLIC AÏOLI

MAKES 8 SERVINGS

PORK

- 2 pork tenderloins (1 pound each)
- Juice of 2 lemons
- 1 tablespoon olive oil
- ½ teaspoon dried rosemary
- Paprika to taste
- Salt and black pepper

AÏOLI

- ½ cup mayonnaise
- 2 tablespoons olive oil
- 2 tablespoons Dijon mustard
- 1 clove garlic, minced
- ⅛ teaspoon salt

1 Preheat oven to 425°F. Place tenderloins in 13×9-inch baking pan; pour lemon juice over top. Drizzle pork with 1 tablespoon oil; sprinkle with rosemary, paprika, salt and pepper. Let stand 15 minutes to marinate.

2 Meanwhile, combine aïoli ingredients in small bowl; cover with plastic wrap and refrigerate until ready to serve.

3 Tuck under thin end of pork. Bake 25 minutes or until barely pink in center (155°F). *Do not overcook.* Remove from oven and let stand 5 minutes. Transfer pork to cutting board; thinly slice.

4 Arrange pork on serving platter. Drizzle pan juices over pork. Serve warm with aïoli.

SERVING SUGGESTION

Serve with roasted brussels sprouts and mashed cauliflower (page 72).

NUTRIENTS PER SERVING (SERVING SIZE: ⅛ OF TOTAL RECIPE)

CALORIES 260   **TOTAL FAT** 18g   **CARBS** 1g   **NET CARBS** 1g   **DIETARY FIBER** 0g   **PROTEIN** 24g

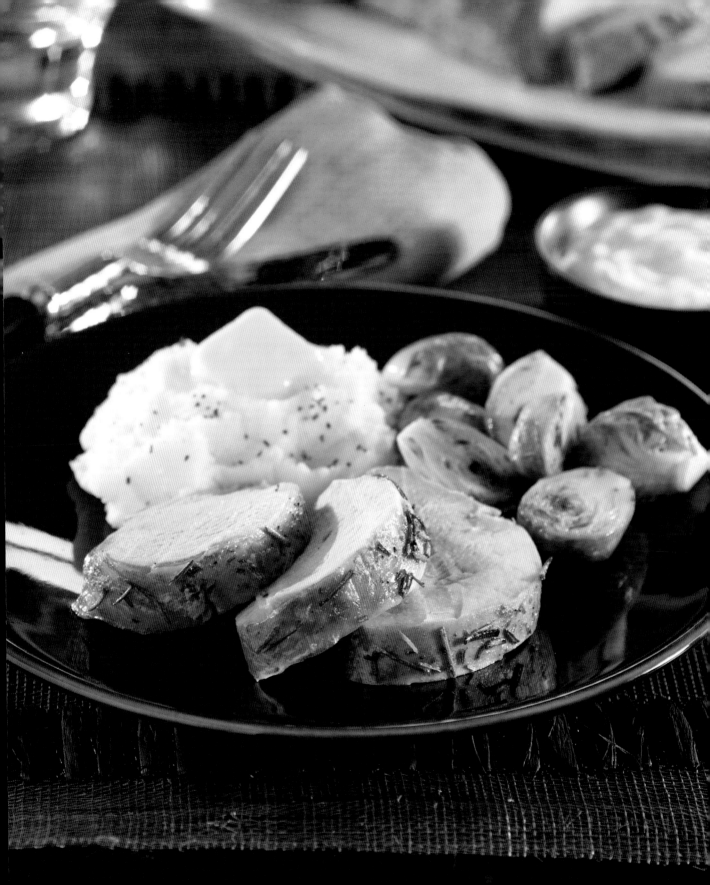

GRILLED STRIP STEAKS WITH CHIMICHURRI

MAKES 4 SERVINGS

4 bone-in strip steaks (8 ounces each), about 1 inch thick

1¼ teaspoons salt, divided

¾ teaspoon ground cumin

¼ teaspoon plus ⅛ teaspoon black pepper, divided

½ cup packed fresh basil leaves

⅓ cup extra virgin olive oil

¼ cup packed fresh parsley

2 tablespoons packed fresh cilantro

2 tablespoons fresh lemon juice

1 clove garlic

½ teaspoon grated orange peel

¼ teaspoon ground coriander

1 Prepare grill for direct cooking. Oil grid. Sprinkle both sides of steaks with ¾ teaspoon salt, cumin and ¼ teaspoon pepper.

2 Grill steaks, covered, over medium-high heat 8 to 10 minutes for medium rare or to desired doneness, turning once.

3 Meanwhile for chimchurri, place basil, oil, parsley, cilantro, lemon juice, garlic, remaining ½ teaspoon salt, orange peel, coriander and remaining ¼ teaspoon pepper in food processor or blender container; process until minced.

NUTRIENTS PER SERVING (SERVING SIZE: 1 STEAK WITH ABOUT ¼ CUP CHIMICHURRI)

CALORIES 630 **TOTAL FAT** 50g **CARBS** 1g **NET CARBS** 1g **DIETARY FIBER** 0g **PROTEIN** 43g

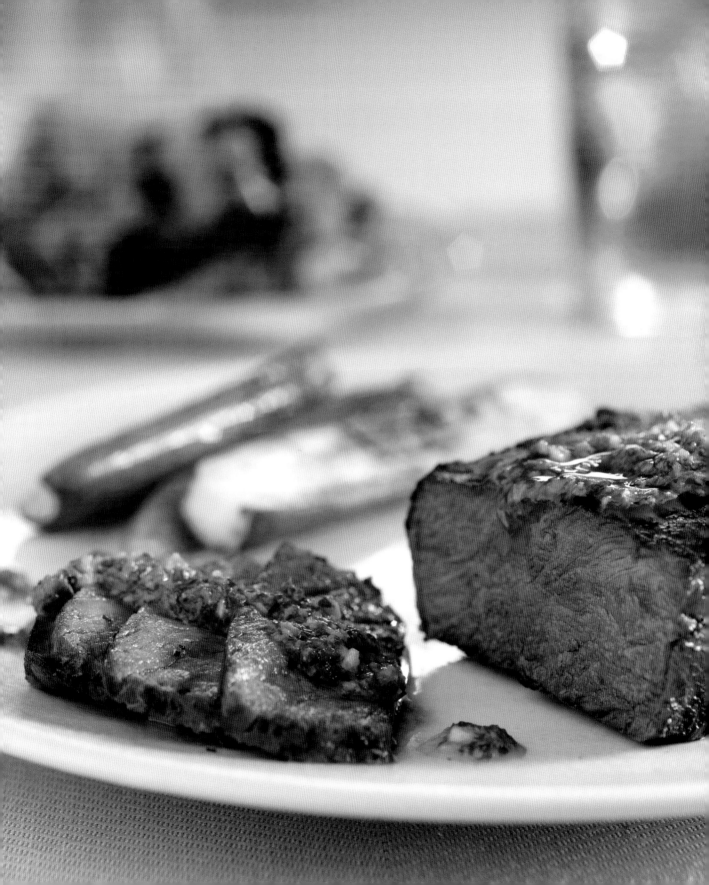

GREEK-STYLE BEEF KABOBS

MAKES 4 SERVINGS

1 pound boneless beef top sirloin steak (1 inch thick), cut into 16 pieces

¼ cup keto Italian salad dressing

3 tablespoons fresh lemon juice, divided

1 tablespoon dried oregano

1 tablespoon Worcestershire sauce

2 teaspoons dried basil

1 teaspoon grated lemon peel

⅛ teaspoon red pepper flakes

1 large green bell pepper, cut into 16 pieces

16 cherry tomatoes

2 teaspoons olive oil

⅛ teaspoon salt

1 Combine beef, salad dressing, 2 tablespoons lemon juice, oregano, Worcestershire, basil, lemon peel and red pepper flakes in large resealable food storage bag. Seal bag; turn to coat. Marinate in refrigerator at least 8 hours or overnight, turning occasionally.

2 Preheat broiler. Remove beef from marinade; reserve marinade. Thread four 10-inch skewers with beef, alternating with bell pepper and tomatoes. Spray rimmed baking sheet or broiler pan with nonstick cooking spray. Brush kabobs with marinade; place on baking sheet. Discard remaining marinade. Broil kabobs 3 minutes. Turn over; broil 2 minutes or until desired doneness. *Do not overcook.* Remove skewers to serving platter.

3 Add remaining 1 tablespoon lemon juice, oil and salt to pan drippings on baking sheet; stir well, scraping up browned bits from bottom of pan. Pour juices over kabobs.

NUTRIENTS PER SERVING (SERVING SIZE: 1 KABOB)

CALORIES 193	**TOTAL FAT** 8g	**CARBS** 5g	**NET CARBS** 4g	**DIETARY FIBER** 1g	**PROTEIN** 25g

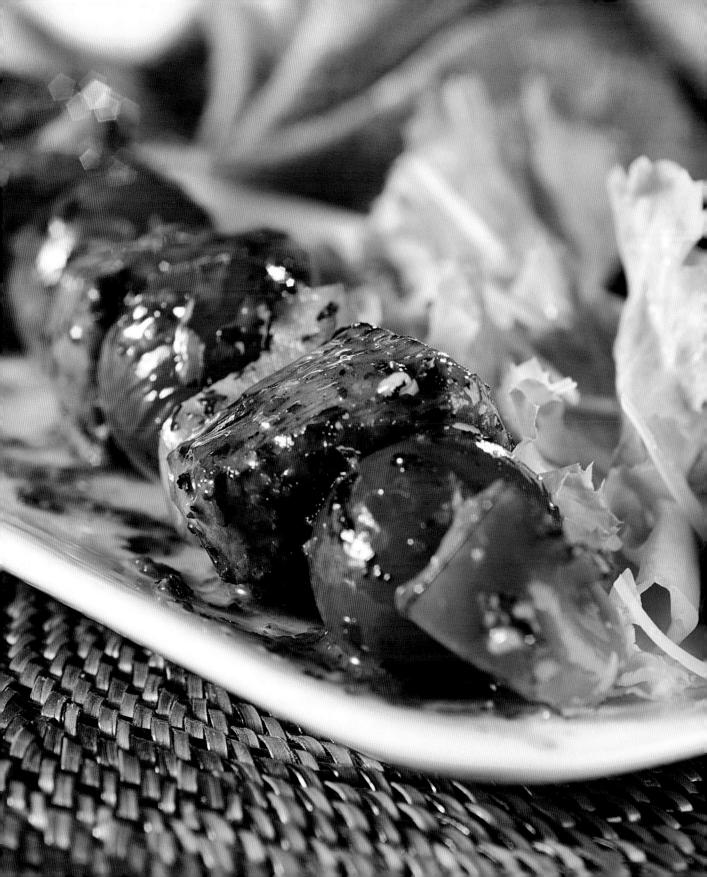

RIB EYE STEAKS WITH CHILI BUTTER

MAKES 4 SERVINGS

½ cup (1 stick) butter, softened

2 teaspoons chili powder

1 teaspoon minced garlic

1 teaspoon Dijon mustard

⅛ teaspoon ground red pepper or chipotle chile pepper

1 teaspoon black pepper

4 beef rib eye steaks

Salt

1 Beat butter, chili powder, garlic, mustard and red pepper in medium bowl until smooth. Place mixture on sheet of waxed paper. Roll mixture back and forth into 6-inch log using waxed paper. If butter is too soft, refrigerate up to 30 minutes. Wrap with waxed paper; refrigerate at least 1 hour or up to 2 days.

2 Prepare grill for direct cooking. Rub black pepper evenly over both sides of steaks; season with salt.

3 Place steaks on grid over medium-high heat. Grill, covered, 8 to 10 minutes or until desired doneness, turning occasionally. Slice chili butter; serve with steak.

NUTRIENTS PER SERVING (SERVING SIZE: 1 STEAK AND 2 TABLESPOONS CHILI BUTTER)

CALORIES 500   **TOTAL FAT** 37g   **CARBS** 2g   **NET CARBS** 1g   **DIETARY FIBER** 1g   **PROTEIN** 40g

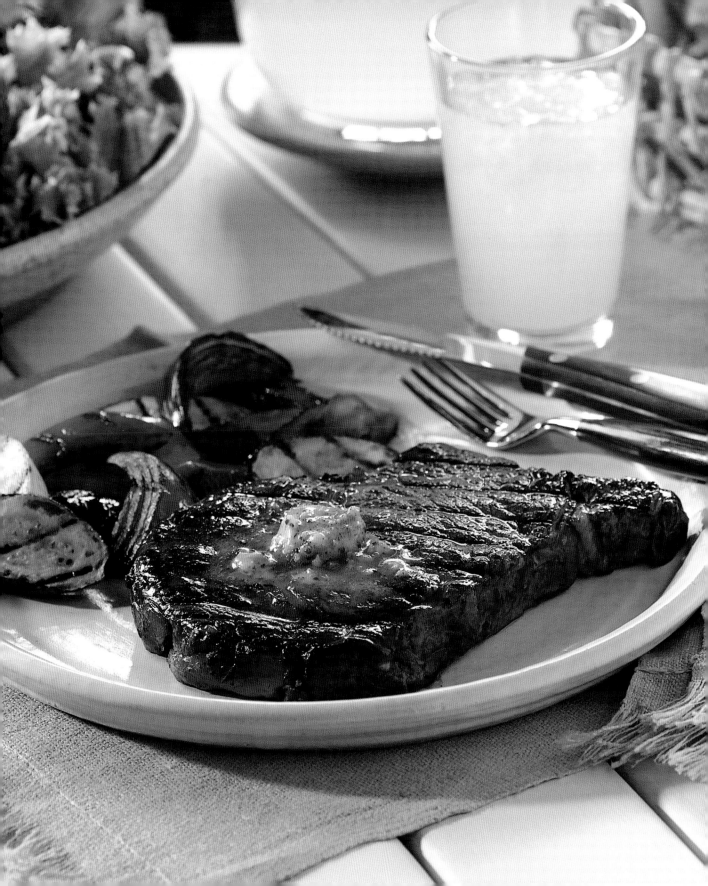

CHINESE PEPPERCORN BEEF

MAKES 4 SERVINGS

- 2 teaspoons whole black and pink peppercorns*
- 2 teaspoons coriander seeds
- 1 tablespoon mild olive oil
- 1 boneless beef top sirloin steak, about 1¼ inches thick (1¼ pounds)
- 2 teaspoons dark sesame oil
- ½ cup thinly sliced shallots or sweet onion
- ½ cup beef broth
- 2 tablespoons soy sauce
- 1 tablespoon dry sherry
- 2 tablespoons thinly sliced green onion or chopped fresh cilantro

You may use all black peppercorns if preferred.

1 Place peppercorns and coriander seeds in small resealable food storage bag; seal bag. Coarsely crush spices using meat mallet or bottom of heavy saucepan. Brush olive oil over both sides of steak; sprinkle with peppercorn mixture, pressing lightly.

2 Heat large heavy skillet over medium-high heat. Add steak; cook 4 minutes without moving or until seared on bottom. Reduce heat to medium; turn steak and continue cooking 3 to 4 minutes for medium rare or until desired doneness. Transfer steak to cutting board; tent with foil and let stand while preparing sauce.

3 Add sesame oil to same skillet; heat over medium heat. Add shallots; cook and stir 3 minutes. Add broth, soy sauce and sherry; simmer about 5 minutes. Carve steak crosswise into thin slices. Spoon sauce over steak; sprinkle with green onion.

NUTRIENTS PER SERVING (SERVING SIZE: 4 OUNCES STEAK AND ¼ CUP SAUCE)

CALORIES 330   **TOTAL FAT** 14g   **CARBS** 4g   **NET CARBS** 3g   **DIETARY FIBER** 1g   **PROTEIN** 43g

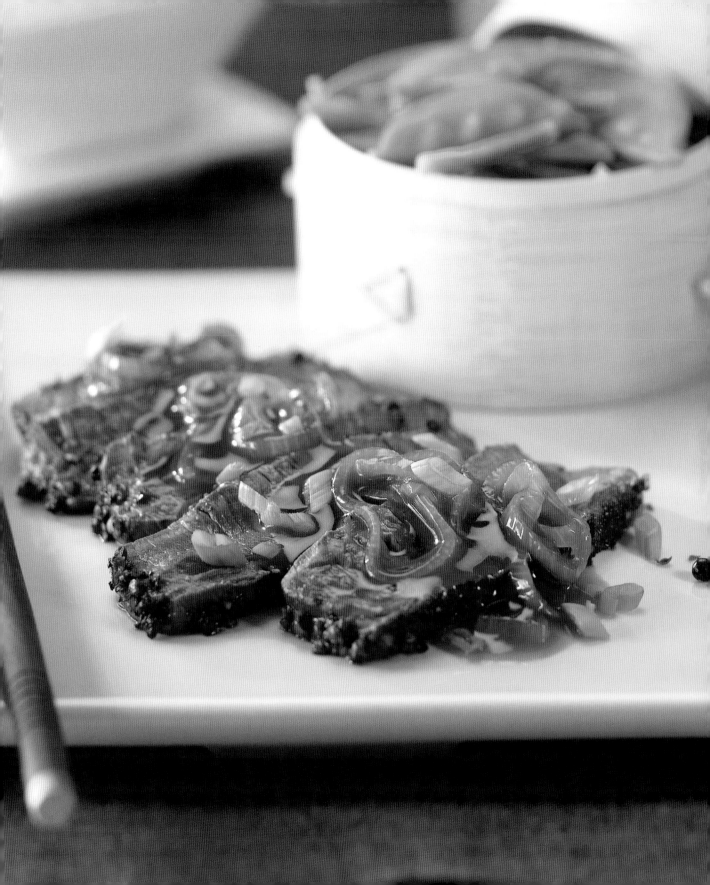

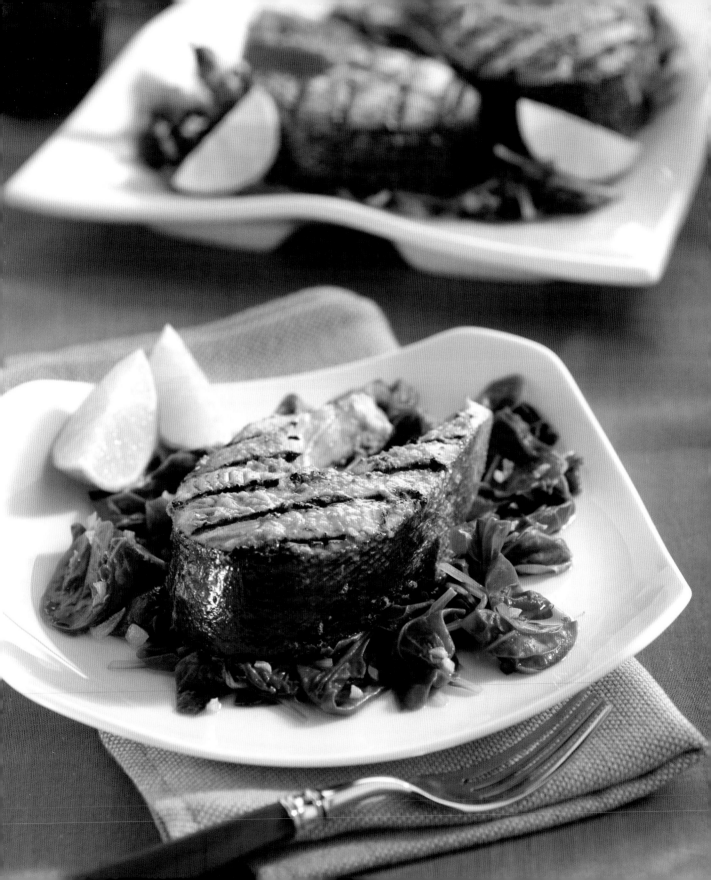

FISH
AND SEAFOOD

GRILLED FIVE-SPICE FISH WITH GARLIC SPINACH

MAKES 4 SERVINGS

1½ teaspoons grated lime peel

3 tablespoons fresh lime juice

4 teaspoons minced fresh ginger

½ to 1 teaspoon Chinese five-spice powder

½ teaspoon salt

⅛ teaspoon black pepper

2 teaspoons mild olive oil, divided

1 pound salmon steaks

8 ounces fresh baby spinach leaves (about 8 cups lightly packed), washed

2 cloves garlic, minced

1 Combine lime peel, lime juice, ginger, five-spice powder, salt, pepper and 1 teaspoon oil in 2-quart dish. Add salmon; turn to coat. Cover and refrigerate 2 to 3 hours.

2 Combine spinach, garlic and remaining 1 teaspoon oil in 3-quart microwavable dish; toss to blend. Cover; microwave on HIGH 2 minutes or until spinach is wilted. Drain; keep warm.

3 Meanwhile, prepare grill for direct cooking over medium-high heat.

4 Remove salmon from marinade and place on oiled grid. Brush salmon with marinade. Grill salmon, covered, 4 minutes. Turn; brush with marinade and grill 4 minutes or until fish just begins to flake when tested with fork. Discard remaining marinade. Serve fish with spinach.

NUTRIENTS PER SERVING (SERVING SIZE: 4 OUNCES SALMON AND ¼ OF SPINACH)

CALORIES 241   **TOTAL FAT** 15g   **CARBS** 3g   **NET CARBS** 2g   **DIETARY FIBER** 1g   **PROTEIN** 24g

CRAB SPINACH SALAD WITH TARRAGON DRESSING

MAKES 4 SERVINGS

12 ounces coarsely flaked cooked crabmeat *or* 2 packages (6 ounces each) frozen crabmeat, thawed and drained

1 cup chopped tomatoes

1 cup sliced cucumber

⅓ cup sliced red onion

¼ cup keto salad dressing or mayonnaise

¼ cup sour cream

¼ cup chopped fresh parsley

2 tablespoons milk

2 teaspoons chopped fresh tarragon *or* ½ teaspoon dried tarragon leaves

1 clove garlic, minced

¼ teaspoon hot pepper sauce

8 cups fresh spinach

1 Combine crabmeat, tomatoes, cucumber and onion in medium bowl. Combine salad dressing, sour cream, parsley, milk, tarragon, garlic and hot pepper sauce in small bowl.

2 Line four salad plates with spinach. Place crabmeat mixture on spinach; drizzle with dressing.

NUTRIENTS PER SERVING
(SERVING SIZE: 1 CUP SALAD, 1¼ TABLESPOONS DRESSING AND 2 CUPS SPINACH)

CALORIES 170　　**TOTAL FAT** 4g　　**CARBS** 14g　　**NET CARBS** 10g　　**DIETARY FIBER** 4g　　**PROTEIN** 22g

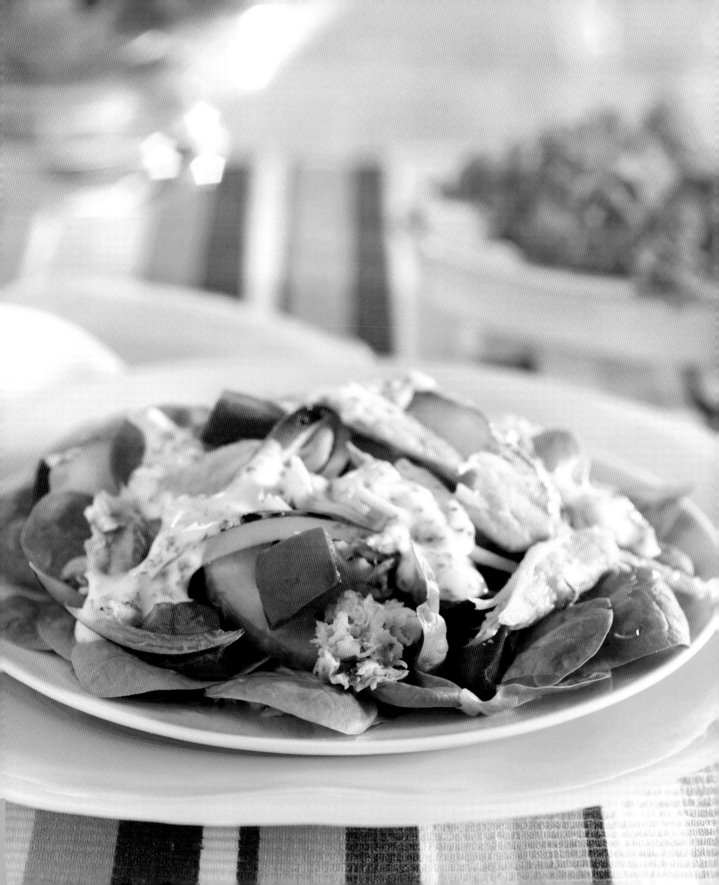

SALMON STEAKS AND ASPARAGUS WITH CILANTRO PESTO

MAKES 4 SERVINGS

1 cup loosely packed fresh cilantro leaves

1 clove garlic, minced

2 tablespoons grated Parmesan cheese

1 tablespoon pine nuts or slivered almonds

3 tablespoons olive oil, divided

2 tablespoons lemon juice, divided

3 teaspoons water
   Salt and black pepper

1 pound asparagus, trimmed

4 salmon steaks (6 ounces each)

1 Spray grid with nonstick cooking spray; prepare grill for direct cooking.

2 For pesto, combine cilantro, garlic, Parmesan, pine nuts, 1 tablespoon oil and 1 tablespoon lemon juice in food processor; process until almost smooth, adding 1 teaspoon water at a time if necessary, until consistency is thick but spreadable. Taste and season with salt and pepper.

3 Bring 1 inch of water to a simmer in large skillet; add 1 teaspoon salt. Add asparagus; cook 3 to 4 minutes or until crisp-tender. Drain and place in serving dish.

4 Meanwhile, sprinkle both sides of salmon with remaining 1 tablespoon lemon juice and brush with remaining 2 tablespoons oil; season with salt and pepper. Grill over medium-high heat about 10 minutes or until fish flakes easily when tested with fork, turning once.

5 Serve salmon with asparagus and pesto.

NUTRIENTS PER SERVING
(SERVING SIZE: 1 SALMON STEAK, ¼ OF ASPARAGUS AND 1 TABLESPOON PESTO)

CALORIES	TOTAL FAT	CARBS	NET CARBS	DIETARY FIBER	PROTEIN
530	39g	7g	4g	3g	40g

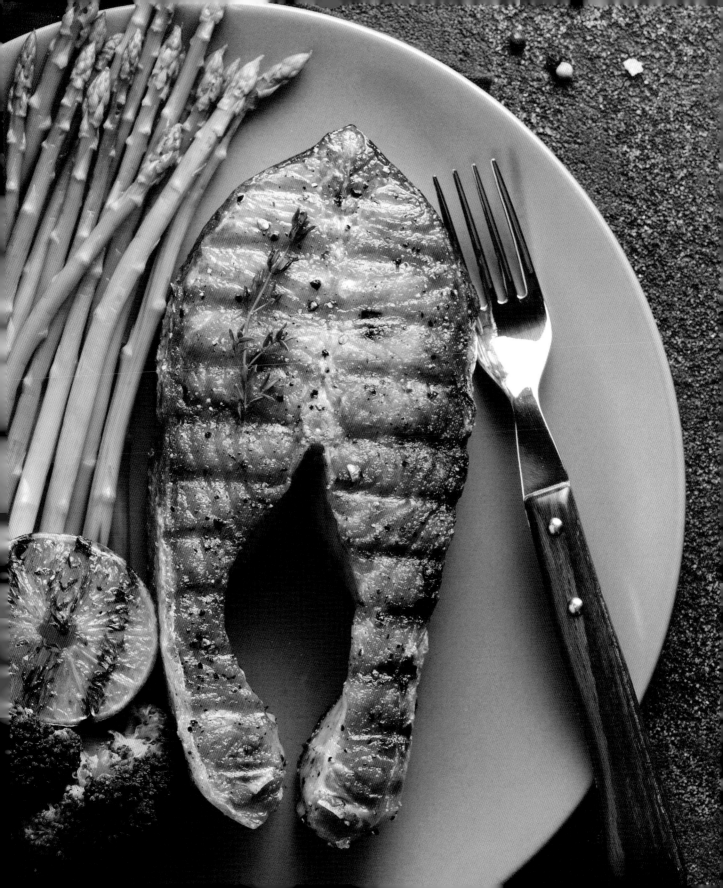

SHRIMP GAZPACHO

MAKES 2 SERVINGS

8 ounces medium shrimp, peeled and deveined

⅛ teaspoon salt

⅛ teaspoon black pepper

1 teaspoon olive oil

3 plum tomatoes, chopped (about 1½ cups)

¼ small red onion, chopped

1 clove garlic, chopped

¼ cucumber, peeled and chopped

¼ cup finely chopped jarred roasted red peppers, divided

¾ cup tomato juice

1 tablespoon red wine vinegar

1 Season shrimp with salt and black pepper. Heat oil in medium nonstick skillet over high heat. Add shrimp; cook 3 minutes or until browned on both sides and opaque in center. Transfer to plate.

2 Combine tomatoes, onion, garlic, cucumber and half of roasted peppers in food processor; process until blended. Add tomato juice and vinegar; process until smooth.

3 Divide tomato mixture among bowls; top with shrimp and remaining roasted peppers.

NUTRIENTS PER SERVING (SERVING SIZE: 1½ CUPS)

CALORIES 150   **TOTAL FAT** 4g   **CARBS** 12g   **NET CARBS** 10g   **DIETARY FIBER** 2g   **PROTEIN** 18g

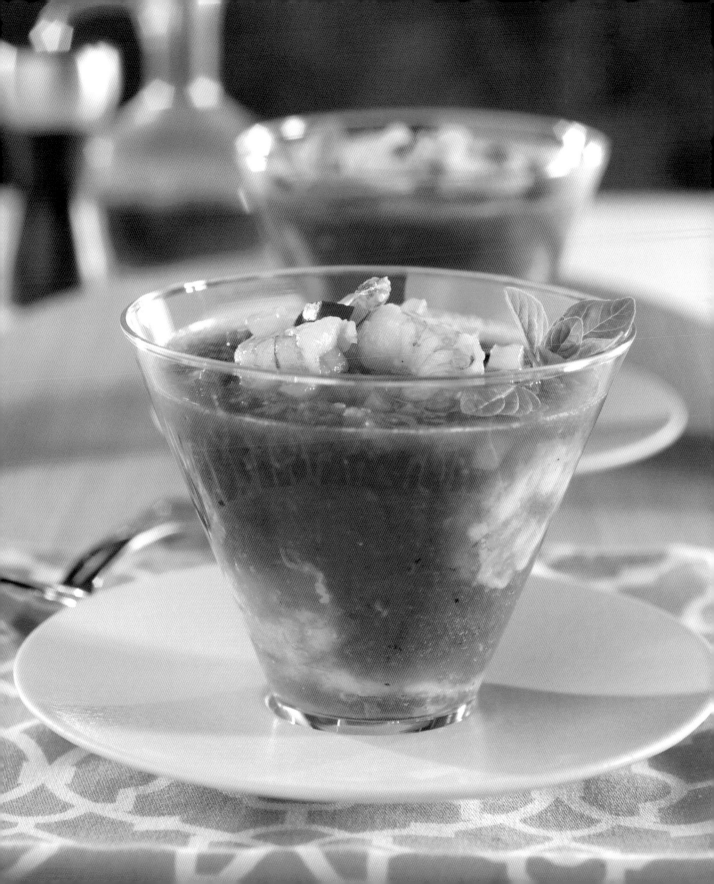

SOY-MARINATED SALMON

MAKES 4 SERVINGS

¼ cup lime juice

¼ cup soy sauce

1 tablespoon grated fresh ginger

1 tablespoon minced garlic

¼ teaspoon black pepper

4 salmon fillets (7 to 8 ounces each)

2 tablespoons minced green onion

1 Combine lime juice, soy sauce, ginger, garlic and pepper in medium bowl; mix well. Reserve ¼ cup mixture for serving; set aside. Place salmon in large resealable food storage bag. Pour remaining mixture over salmon; seal bag and turn to coat. Marinate in refrigerator 2 to 4 hours, turning occasionally.

2 Prepare grill or preheat broiler. Remove salmon from marinade; discard marinade.

3 Grill or broil salmon 10 minutes or until fish begins to flake when tested with fork. (To broil, place salmon on foil-lined baking sheet sprayed with nonstick cooking spray.) Brush with some of reserved marinade mixture; sprinkle with green onion.

NUTRIENTS PER SERVING (SERVING SIZE: ¼ OF TOTAL RECIPE)

CALORIES 440 **TOTAL FAT** 27g **CARBS** 3g **NET CARBS** 3g **DIETARY FIBER** 0g **PROTEIN** 45g

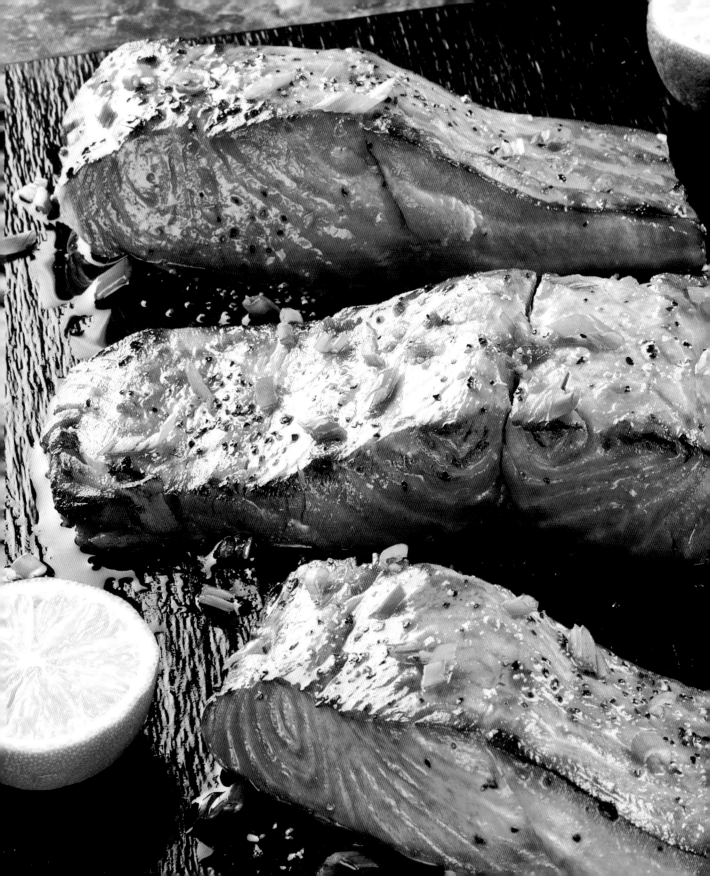

BAKED FISH WITH THAI PESTO

MAKES 6 SERVINGS

1 to 2 jalapeño peppers,
   coarsely chopped

1 lemon

4 green onions, thinly
   sliced

2 tablespoons chopped
   fresh ginger

3 cloves garlic, minced

1½ cups lightly packed
   fresh basil leaves

1 cup lightly packed
   fresh cilantro leaves

¼ cup lightly packed
   fresh mint leaves

¼ cup unsalted roasted
   peanuts

2 tablespoons
   unsweetened
   shredded coconut

½ cup mild olive oil

2 pounds boneless
   fish fillets (such as
   salmon, halibut, cod
   or orange roughy)

Lemon and cucumber
   slices (optional)

1 Place jalapeños in food processor.

2 Grate peel of lemon. Juice lemon to measure
2 tablespoons. Add peel and juice to food processor.

3 Add green onions, ginger, garlic, basil, cilantro, mint,
peanuts and coconut to food processor; process until
finely chopped. With motor running, slowly pour in oil;
process until mixed.

4 Preheat oven to 375°F. Rinse fish and pat dry with paper
towels. Place fillets on lightly oiled baking sheet. Spread
solid thin layer of pesto over each fillet.

5 Bake 10 minutes or until fish begins to flake when tested
with fork and is just opaque in center. Transfer fish to
serving platter with wide spatula. Garnish with lemon and
cucumber slices.

NUTRIENTS PER SERVING (SERVING SIZE: ⅙ OF TOTAL RECIPE)

CALORIES	TOTAL FAT	CARBS	NET CARBS	DIETARY FIBER	PROTEIN
530	43g	4g	2g	2g	33g

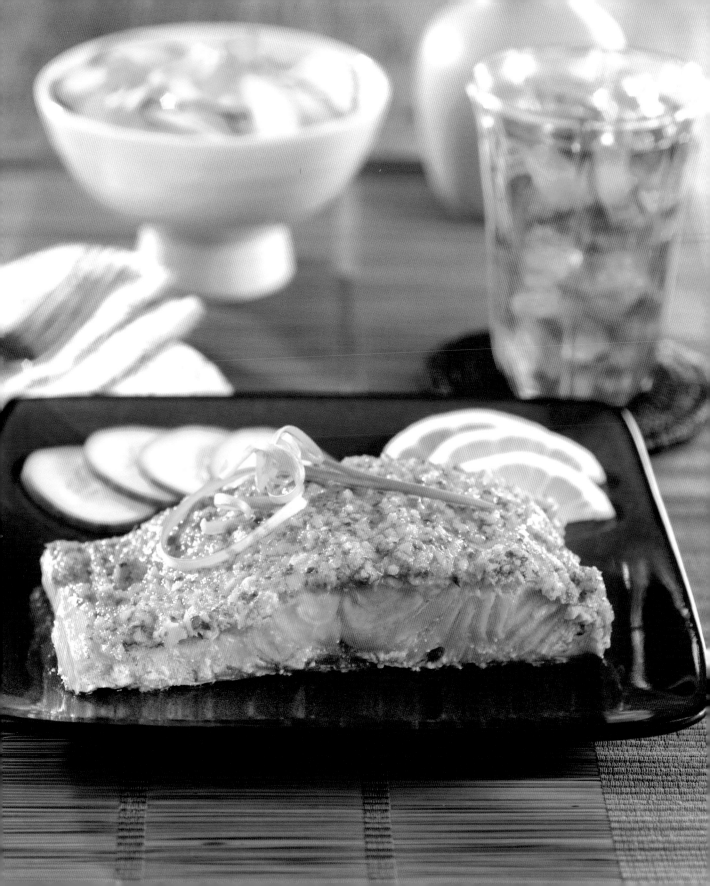

TUNA TERIYAKI

MAKES 4 SERVINGS

4 fresh tuna steaks*
    (about 1½ pounds)
¼ cup soy sauce
2 tablespoons sake
½ teaspoon minced fresh
    ginger
¼ teaspoon minced
    garlic
1½ tablespoons mild
    olive oil
2 limes, cut in half
    Pickled ginger
    (optional)

*Salmon, halibut or
swordfish can be
substituted for the tuna.

1 Place tuna in shallow dish. Whisk soy sauce, sake, ginger and garlic in small bowl until smooth. Pour over tuna. Cover and marinate in refrigerator 40 minutes, turning frequently.

2 Drain tuna, reserving marinade. Heat oil in large skillet over medium heat. Add tuna; cook 2 to 3 minutes or until light brown. Turn over; cook 2 to 3 minutes or just until opaque.

3 Reduce heat to medium-low. Pour reserved marinade over tuna. Add limes, cut side down, to skillet. Cook 1 to 1½ minutes or until tuna is coated with sauce and sauce is bubbly, carefully turning tuna once. Serve with limes and pickled ginger, if desired.

NUTRIENTS PER SERVING (SERVING SIZE: ¼ OF TOTAL RECIPE)

CALORIES 310	TOTAL FAT 14g	CARBS 2g	NET CARBS 2g	DIETARY FIBER 0g	PROTEIN 41g

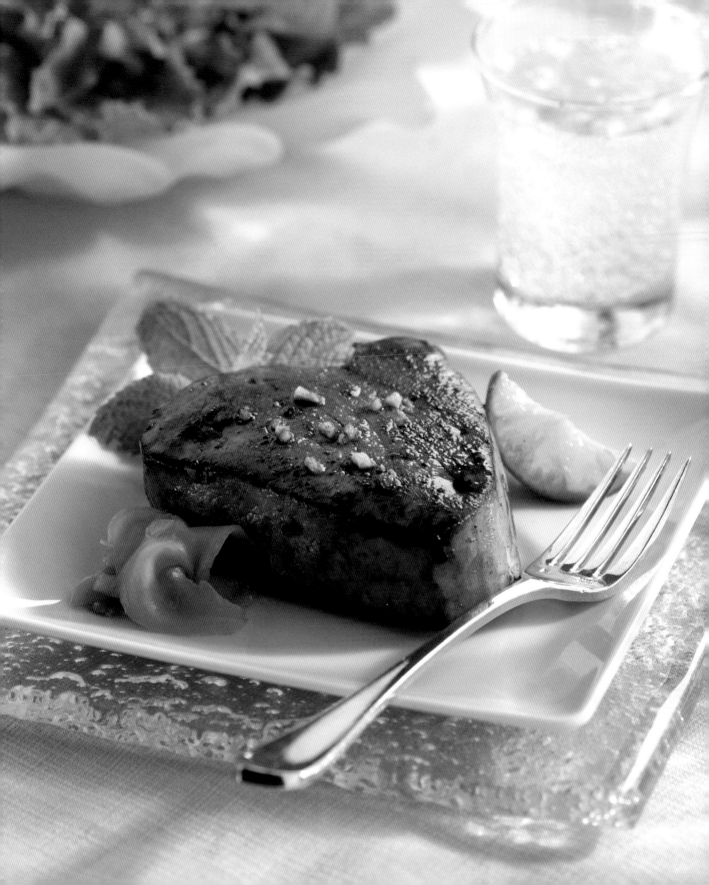

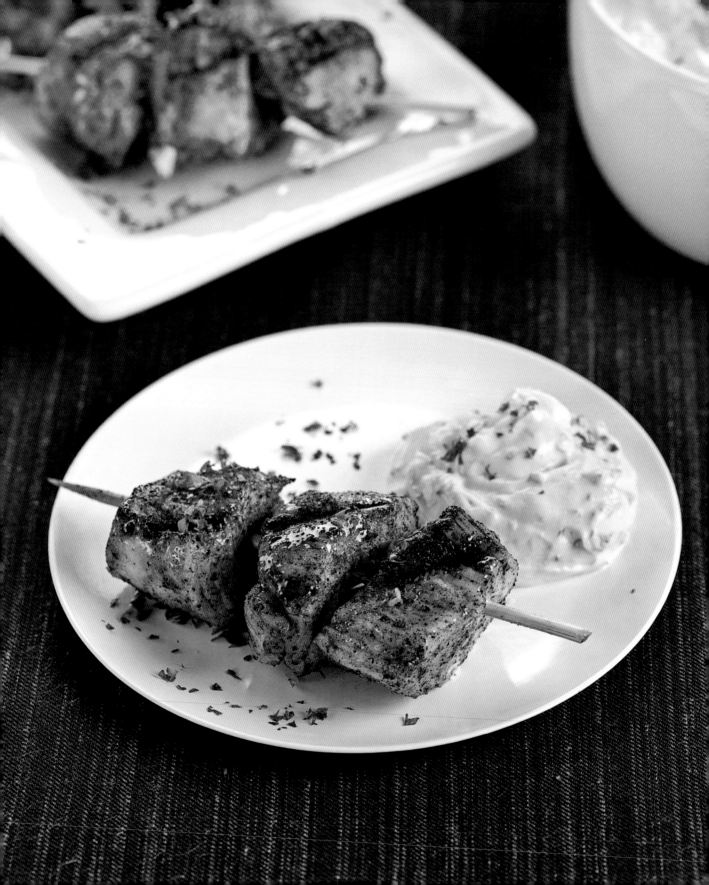

CHICKEN AND TURKEY

SPICED CHICKEN SKEWERS WITH YOGURT-TAHINI SAUCE

MAKES 8 SERVINGS

1 cup plain Greek yogurt

¼ cup chopped fresh parsley, plus additional for garnish

¼ cup tahini

2 tablespoons lemon juice

1 clove garlic

¾ teaspoon salt, divided

1 tablespoon olive oil

2 teaspoons garam masala

1 pound boneless skinless chicken breasts, cut into 1-inch pieces

1 Soak eight 6-inch bamboo skewers in cold water 20 minutes. Spray grid with nonstick cooking spray. Prepare grill for direct cooking.

2 For sauce, combine yogurt, ¼ cup parsley, tahini, lemon juice, garlic and ¼ teaspoon salt in food processor or blender; process until smooth.

3 Combine oil, garam masala and remaining ½ teaspoon salt in medium bowl. Add chicken; toss to coat. Thread on skewers.

4 Grill chicken skewers over medium-high heat 10 minutes or until chicken is no longer pink, turning once. Serve with sauce. Garnish with additional parsley.

NUTRIENTS PER SERVING (SERVING SIZE: 1 SKEWER WITH ABOUT 2 TABLESPOONS SAUCE)

CALORIES 145 **TOTAL FAT** 7g **CARBS** 4g **NET CARBS** 4g **DIETARY FIBER** 0g **PROTEIN** 16g

TURKEY AND VEGGIE MEATBALLS WITH FENNEL

MAKES 6 SERVINGS

1 pound ground turkey

½ cup finely chopped green onions

½ cup finely chopped green bell pepper

⅓ cup almond flour

¼ cup shredded carrot (optional)

¼ cup grated Parmesan cheese

2 egg whites

2 tablespoons whipping cream

2 cloves garlic, minced

½ teaspoon Italian seasoning

¼ teaspoon fennel seeds

¼ teaspoon salt

⅛ teaspoon red pepper flakes (optional)

1 tablespoon extra virgin olive oil

Marinara sauce, heated (optional)

1 Combine turkey, green onions, bell pepper, almond flour, carrot, if desired, Parmesan, egg whites, cream and garlic in large bowl. Combine Italian seasoning, fennel, salt and red pepper flakes, if desired, in small bowl. Add to turkey mixture; mix well. Shape into 36 (1-inch) balls.

2 Heat oil in large nonstick skillet over medium-high heat. Add meatballs; cook 10 to 12 minutes or until no longer pink in center, turning frequently. Serve with marinara sauce, if desired.

SERVING SUGGESTION

To freeze leftover meatballs, cool completely and place in gallon-size resealable food storage bag. Release any excess air from bag and seal. Freeze bag flat for easier storage and faster thawing. This will also allow you to remove as many meatballs as needed without them sticking together. To reheat, place meatballs in a 12×8-inch microwavable dish and cook on HIGH 20 to 30 seconds or until hot.

NUTRIENTS PER SERVING (SERVING SIZE: 6 MEATBALLS)

CALORIES 170   **TOTAL FAT** 8g   **CARBS** 3g   **NET CARBS** 2g   **DIETARY FIBER** 1g   **PROTEIN** 23g

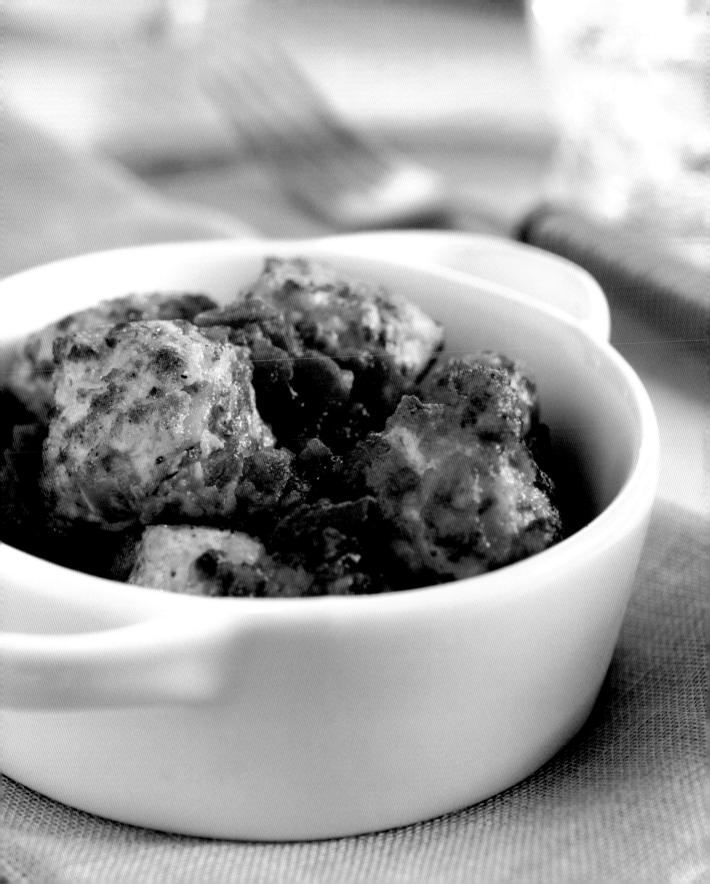

SALSA CHICKEN AND PEPPERS

MAKES 4 SERVINGS

1 tablespoon Mexican seasoning*

4 small boneless skinless chicken breasts (about ¼ pound each) *or* 2 large boneless skinless chicken breasts, cut in half and pounded to 1-inch thickness

1 tablespoon vegetable oil

1 red onion, sliced

1 medium red bell pepper, cut into thin strips

1 medium yellow or green bell pepper, cut into thin strips

½ cup chunky salsa or chipotle salsa

2 tablespoons lime juice

Lime wedges (optional)

If Mexican seasoning is not available, substitute 1 teaspoon chili powder, ½ teaspoon ground cumin, ½ teaspoon salt and ⅛ teaspoon ground red pepper.

1 Sprinkle Mexican seasoning over both sides of chicken; set aside.

2 Heat oil! in large nonstick skillet over medium heat. Add onion; cook 3 minutes, stirring occasionally.

3 Add bell peppers; cook 3 minutes, stirring occasionally. Stir in salsa and lime juice.

4 Push vegetables to edge of skillet. Add chicken to skillet. Cook 5 minutes; turn. Continue to cook 4 minutes or until chicken is no longer pink in center (165°F) and vegetables are tender.

5 Serve chicken over vegetables; garnish with lime wedges.

NUTRIENTS PER SERVING (SERVING SIZE: ¼ OF TOTAL RECIPE)

CALORIES 224 **TOTAL FAT** 8g **CARBS** 11g **NET CARBS** 8g **DIETARY FIBER** 3g **PROTEIN** 27g

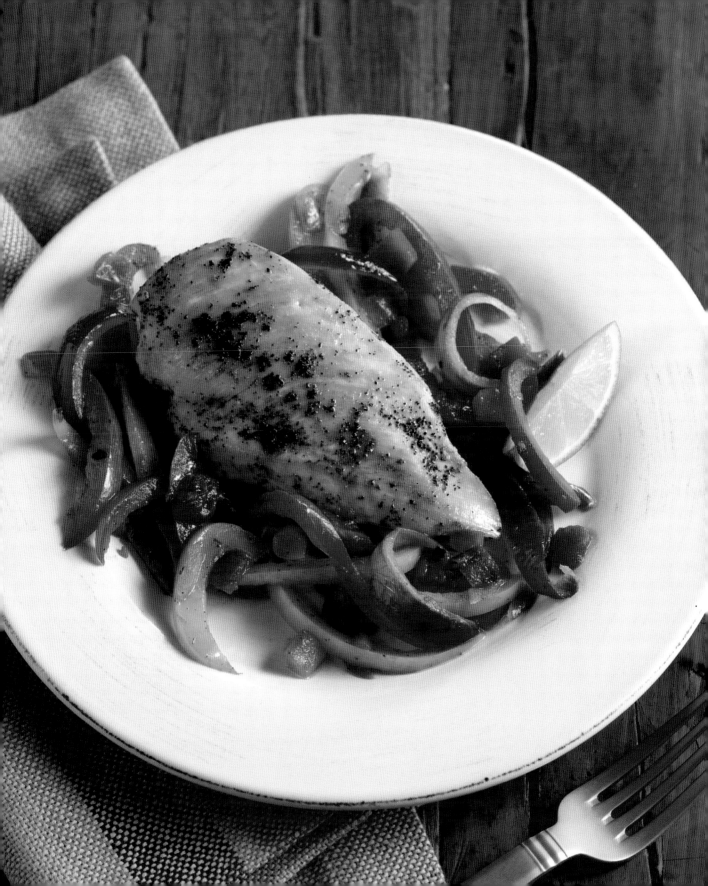

ROASTED ROSEMARY CHICKEN LEGS

MAKES 4 SERVINGS

¼ cup finely chopped onion

2 tablespoons butter, melted

1 tablespoon chopped fresh rosemary leaves *or* 1 teaspoon dried rosemary

½ teaspoon salt

¼ teaspoon black pepper

2 cloves garlic, minced

4 chicken leg quarters (about 1½ pounds)

¼ cup chicken broth or white wine

1 Preheat oven to 375°F.

2 Combine onion, butter, rosemary, salt, pepper and garlic in small bowl; mix well. Gently loosen chicken skin; rub onion mixture under and over skin. Place chicken, skin side up, in small shallow roasting pan. Pour wine over chicken.

3 Roast chicken 50 to 60 minutes or until chicken is browned and cooked through (165°F), basting frequently with pan juices.

NUTRIENTS PER SERVING (SERVING SIZE: ¼ OF TOTAL RECIPE)

CALORIES 263   **TOTAL FAT** 17g   **CARBS** 2g   **NET CARBS** 1g   **DIETARY FIBER** 1g   **PROTEIN** 22g

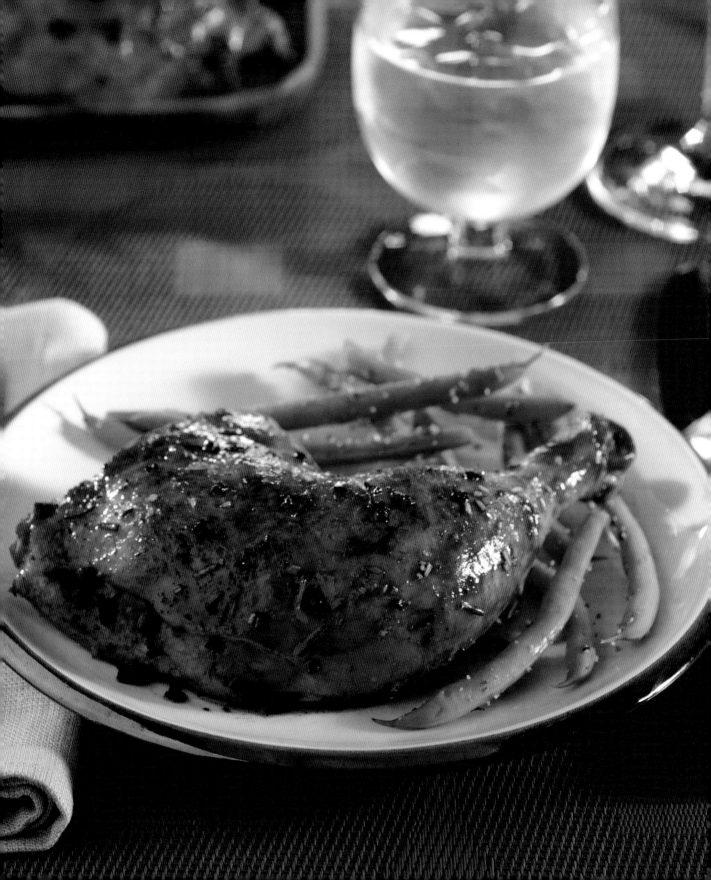

TURKEY TACO BOWLS

MAKES 4 SERVINGS

1 pound ground turkey

1 tablespoon chili powder

1 teaspoon paprika

1 teaspoon ground cumin

½ teaspoon dried oregano

½ teaspoon salt

¼ teaspoon garlic powder

¼ teaspoon onion powder

¾ cup water

1 bag (10 ounces) frozen cauliflower rice

2 cups shredded red cabbage

2 green onions, finely chopped

1 avocado, thinly sliced

2 plum tomatoes, diced

Minced fresh cilantro, sour cream and crumbled cotija cheese

1 Cook turkey in large nonstick skillet over medium-high heat 6 to 8 minutes or until no longer pink, stirring to break up meat. Stir in chili powder, paprika, cumin, oregano, salt, garlic powder, onion powder and water; bring to a boil. Reduce heat to medium-low; simmer 5 minutes, stirring occasionally. Set aside.

2 Heat cauliflower rice according to package directions. Divide among four bowls. Add turkey, cabbage, green onions, avocado and tomatoes. Serve with cilantro, sour cream and cotija cheese.

NUTRIENTS PER SERVING (SERVING SIZE: ¼ OF TOTAL RECIPE)

CALORIES 250   **TOTAL FAT** 9g   **CARBS** 15g   **NET CARBS** 8g   **DIETARY FIBER** 7g   **PROTEIN** 31g

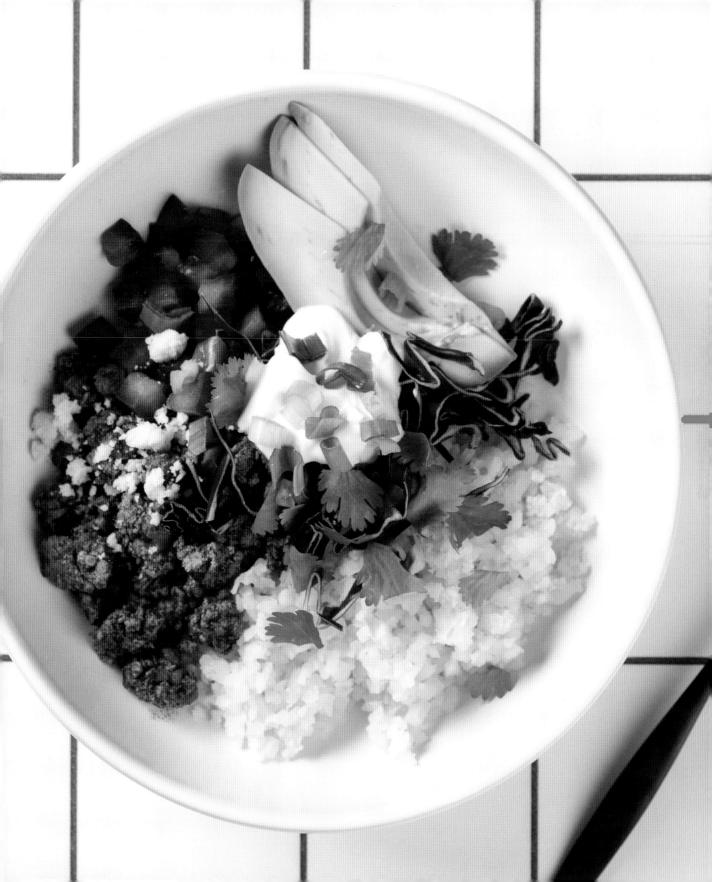

INDIAN-INSPIRED CHICKEN WITH RAITA

MAKES 6 SERVINGS

- 1 cup plain yogurt
- 2 cloves garlic, minced
- 1 teaspoon salt
- 1 teaspoon ground coriander
- 1 teaspoon ground ginger
- ½ teaspoon ground turmeric
- ½ teaspoon ground cinnamon
- ½ teaspoon ground cumin
- ¼ teaspoon ground red pepper
- 1 (5- to 6-pound) chicken, cut into 8 pieces (about 4 pounds chicken parts)

RAITA

- 2 medium cucumbers (about 1 pound), peeled, seeded and thinly sliced
- ⅓ cup plain yogurt
- 2 tablespoons chopped fresh cilantro
- 1 clove garlic, minced
- ¼ teaspoon salt
- ⅛ teaspoon black pepper

1 Mix 1 cup yogurt, 2 cloves garlic, 1 teaspoon salt, coriander, ginger, turmeric, cinnamon, cumin and red pepper in medium bowl. Place chicken in large resealable food storage bag; add yogurt mixture. Seal bag; turn to coat. Marinate in refrigerator 4 to 24 hours, turning occasionally.

2 Preheat broiler. Cover baking sheet with foil. Place chicken on prepared baking sheet; discard marinade. Broil 6 inches from heat source about 30 minutes or until cooked through (165°F), turning once.

3 Meanwhile for raita, combine cucumbers, ⅓ cup yogurt, cilantro, 1 clove garlic, ¼ teaspoon salt and black pepper in small bowl. Serve with chicken.

NUTRIENTS PER SERVING (SERVING SIZE: ⅙ OF TOTAL RECIPE)

CALORIES 625   **TOTAL FAT** 43g   **CARBS** 8g   **NET CARBS** 7g   **DIETARY FIBER** 1g   **PROTEIN** 50g

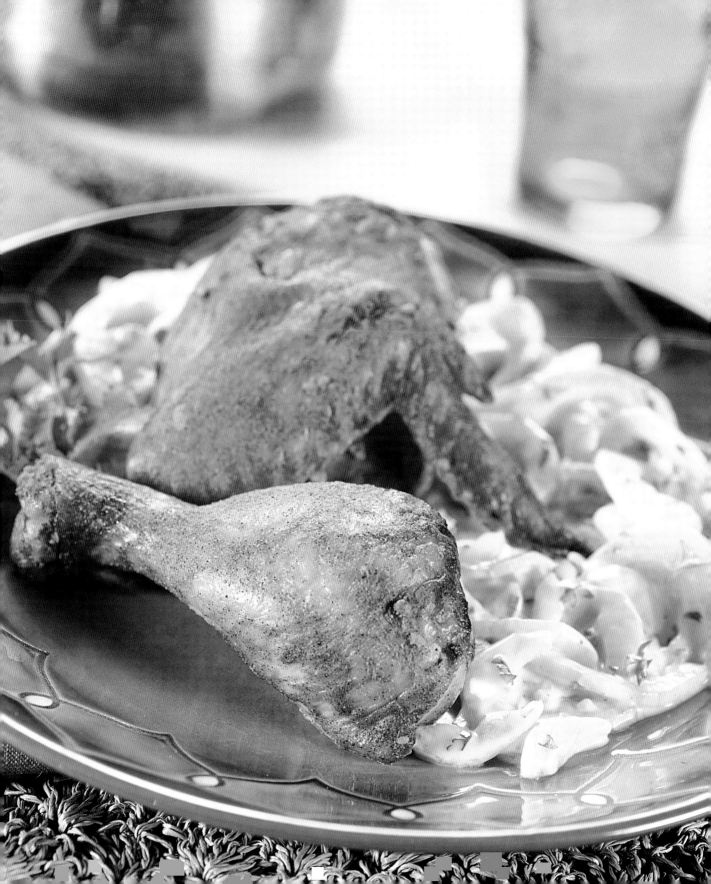

PESTO-STUFFED GRILLED CHICKEN

MAKES 6 SERVINGS

2 cloves garlic, peeled

½ cup packed fresh basil leaves

2 tablespoons pine nuts or walnuts, toasted*

Salt and pepper

5 tablespoons extra virgin olive oil, divided

¼ cup grated Parmesan cheese

1 fresh or thawed frozen roasting chicken or capon (6 to 7 pounds)

2 tablespoons fresh lemon juice

To toast pine nuts, spread in single layer in small heavy skillet. Cook and stir 2 to 3 minutes or until golden brown, stirring frequently.

1 Prepare grill with metal or foil drip pan. Bank briquettes on either side of drip pan for indirect cooking.

2 For pesto, drop garlic through feed tube of food processor with motor running. Add basil, pine nuts and ¼ teaspoon black pepper; process until basil is minced. With motor running, add 3 tablespoons oil in thin, steady stream until smooth paste forms, scraping down side of bowl once. Add cheese; process until well blended. Season with salt to taste.

3 Remove giblets from chicken cavity; reserve for another use. Loosen skin over breast of chicken by pushing fingers between skin and meat, taking care not to tear skin. Do not loosen skin over wings and drumsticks. Using rubber spatula or small spoon, spread pesto under breast skin; massage skin to evenly spread pesto. Combine remaining 2 tablespoons oil and lemon juice in small bowl; brush over chicken skin. Season with salt and pepper. Tuck wings under back; tie legs together with kitchen string.

4 Place chicken, breast side up, on grid directly over drip pan. Grill, covered, over medium-low coals 1 hour 10 minutes to 1 hour 30 minutes or until thermometer inserted into thickest part of thigh not touching bone registers 185°F, adding 4 to 9 briquettes to both sides of the fire after 45 minutes to maintain medium-low coals. Transfer chicken to large cutting board; tent with foil. Let stand 15 minutes before carving.

NUTRIENTS PER SERVING (SERVING SIZE: 4 OUNCES)

CALORIES 280 **TOTAL FAT** 18g **CARBS** 4g **NET CARBS** 4g **DIETARY FIBER** 0g **PROTEIN** 25g

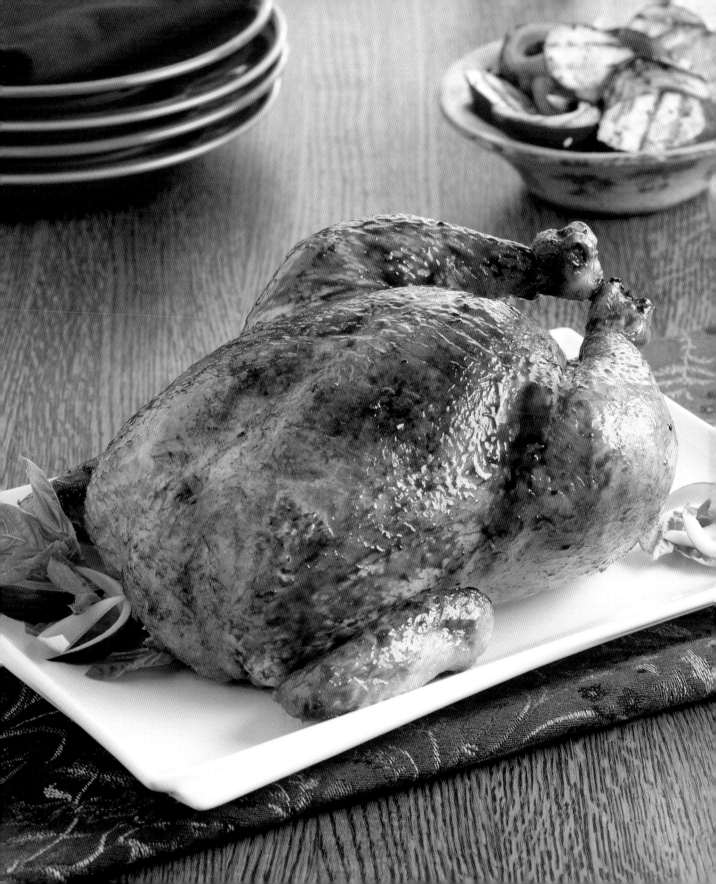

KALE & MUSHROOM STUFFED CHICKEN BREASTS

MAKES 4 SERVINGS

- 3 teaspoons olive oil, divided
- 1 cup coarsely chopped mushrooms
- 2 cups thinly sliced kale
- 1 tablespoon fresh lemon juice
- ½ teaspoon salt, divided
- 4 boneless skinless chicken breasts (about 4 ounces each)
- ¼ cup crumbled feta cheese
- ¼ teaspoon black pepper

1 Heat 1 teaspoon oil in large skillet over medium-high heat. Add mushrooms; cook and stir 5 minutes or until beginning to brown. Add kale; cook and stir 8 minutes or until wilted. Sprinkle with lemon juice and ¼ teaspoon salt. Transfer to small bowl. Let stand 5 to 10 minutes to cool slightly.

2 Meanwhile, place chicken breasts between sheets of plastic wrap. Pound with meat mallet or rolling pin to about ½-inch thickness.

3 Gently stir feta into mushroom and kale mixture. Spoon ¼ cup mixture down center of each chicken breast. Roll up to enclose filling; secure with toothpicks. Sprinkle with remaining ¼ teaspoon salt and pepper.

4 Wipe out same skillet with paper towels. Add remaining 2 teaspoons oil to skillet; heat over medium heat. Add chicken; brown on all sides. Cover and cook 5 minutes per side or until no longer pink. Remove toothpicks before serving.

NUTRIENTS PER SERVING (SERVING SIZE: ¼ OF TOTAL RECIPE)

CALORIES 192   **TOTAL FAT** 7g   **CARBS** 4g   **NET CARBS** 3g   **DIETARY FIBER** 1g   **PROTEIN** 29g

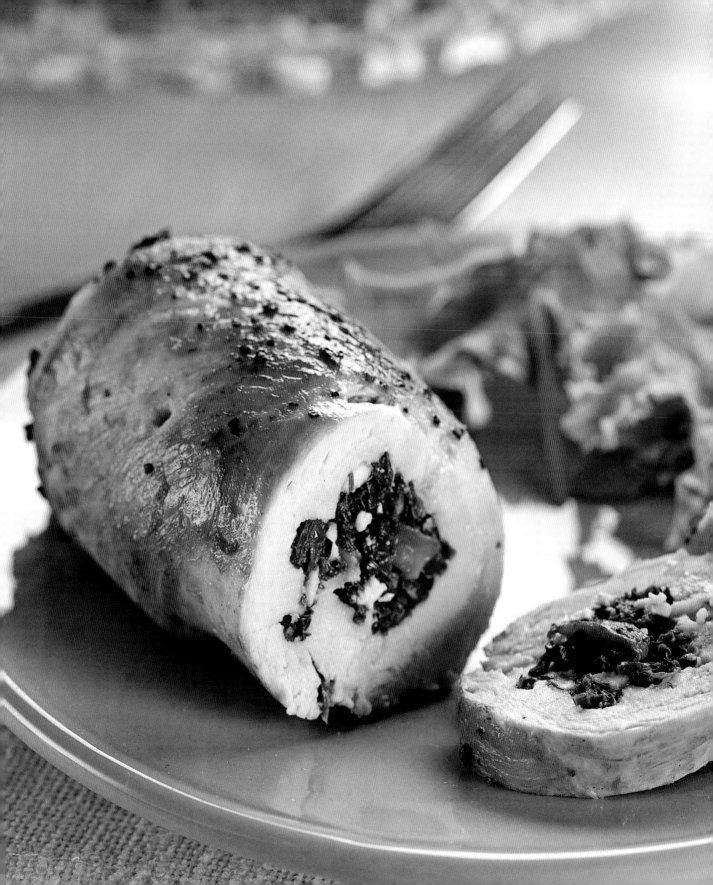

CHICKEN AVOCADO BOATS

MAKES 6 SERVINGS

3 large ripe avocados, cut in half and pitted

6 tablespoons lemon juice

¾ cup mayonnaise

1½ tablespoons grated onion

¼ teaspoon celery salt

¼ teaspoon garlic powder

2 cups diced cooked chicken

Salt and black pepper

½ cup (2 ounces) shredded sharp Cheddar cheese

Minced fresh chives (optional)

1 Preheat oven to 350°F. Sprinkle each avocado half with 1 tablespoon lemon juice; set aside.

2 Combine mayonnaise, onion, celery salt and garlic powder in medium bowl. Stir in chicken; mix well. Season with salt and pepper.

3 Drain any excess lemon juice from avocado halves. Fill avocado halves with chicken mixture; sprinkle with cheese. Arrange filled avocado halves in single layer in baking dish. Pour water into same dish to depth of ½ inch.

4 Bake 15 minutes or until cheese melts. Garnish with chives.

NUTRIENTS PER SERVING (SERVING SIZE: 1 FILLED AVOCADO HALF)

CALORIES 490   **TOTAL FAT** 42g   **CARBS** 11g   **NET CARBS** 4g   **DIETARY FIBER** 7g   **PROTEIN** 20g

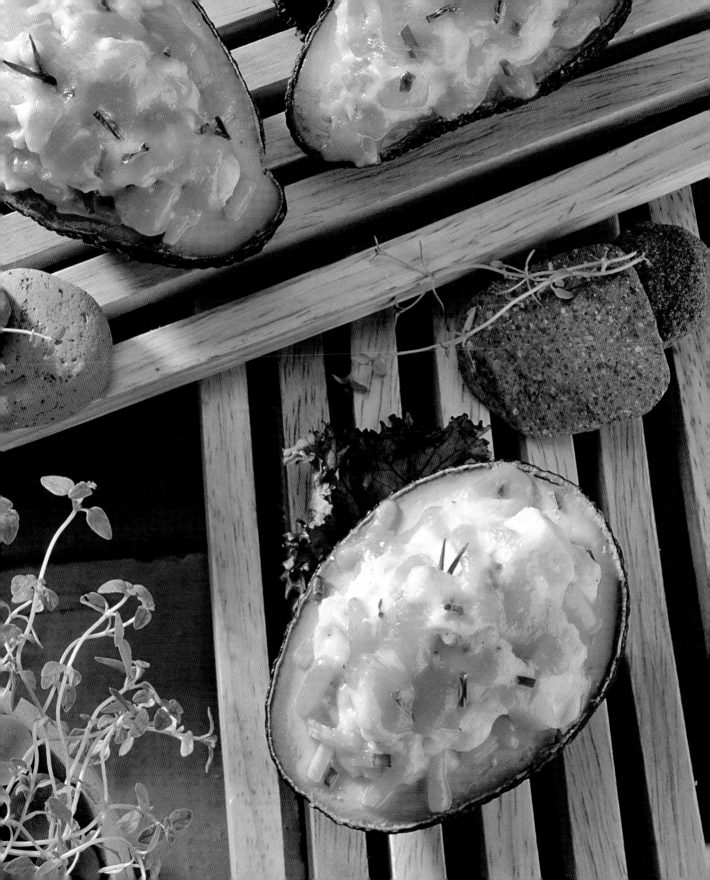

CHICKEN PICCATA
MAKES 4 SERVINGS

3 tablespoons almond
 flour

½ teaspoon salt

¼ teaspoon black pepper

4 small boneless skinless
 chicken breasts
 (4 ounces each)

2 teaspoons olive oil

1 teaspoon butter

2 cloves garlic, minced

¾ cup chicken broth

1 tablespoon fresh
 lemon juice

2 tablespoons chopped
 fresh Italian parsley

1 tablespoon capers,
 drained

1 Combine almond flour, salt and pepper in shallow dish. Reserve 1 tablespoon flour mixture.

2 Pound chicken between waxed paper to ½-inch thickness with flat side of meat mallet or rolling pin. Coat chicken with remaining flour mixture, shaking off excess.

3 Heat oil and butter in large nonstick skillet over medium heat. Add chicken; cook 4 to 5 minutes per side or until no longer pink in center. Transfer to serving platter; cover loosely with foil.

4 Add garlic to same skillet; cook and stir 1 minute. Add reserved flour mixture; cook and stir 1 minute. Add broth and lemon juice; cook 2 minutes or until thickened, stirring frequently. Stir in parsley and capers; spoon sauce over chicken.

NUTRIENTS PER SERVING (SERVING SIZE: ¼ OF TOTAL RECIPE)

CALORIES 194   **TOTAL FAT** 6g   **CARBS** 5g   **NET CARBS** 4g   **DIETARY FIBER** 1g   **PROTEIN** 27g

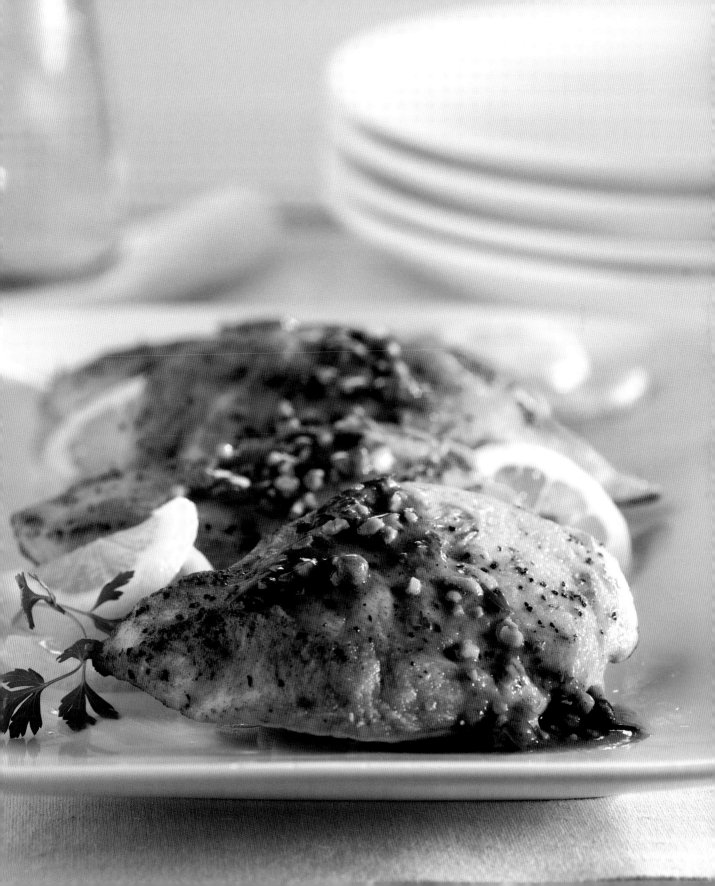

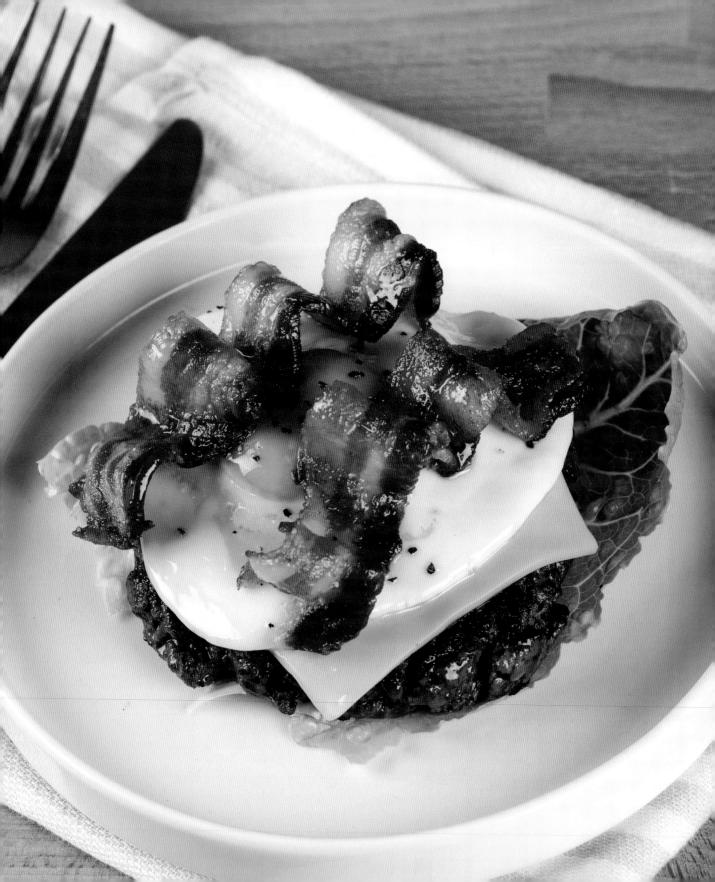

SANDWICHES AND BURGERS

BACON SMASHBURGER
MAKES 4 SERVINGS

4 slices bacon, cut in half
1 pound ground chuck
   Salt and black pepper
4 slices sharp Cheddar
   cheese
4 eggs (optional)
   Lettuce leaves

1 Cook bacon in large skillet over medium-high heat until crisp. Remove from skillet; drain on paper towels. Drain all but 1 tablespoon drippings from skillet.

2 Divide beef into 4 portions and shape lightly into loose balls. Place in same skillet over medium-high heat. Smash with spatula to flatten into thin patties; sprinkle with salt and pepper. Cook 2 to 3 minutes or until edges and bottoms are browned. Flip burgers and top with 1 slice of cheese. Cook 2 to 3 minutes for medium rare or to desired degree of doneness. Transfer to plates.

3 If desired, crack eggs into hot skillet. Cook over medium heat about 3 minutes or until whites are opaque and yolks are desired degree of doneness, flipping once, if desired, for overeasy. Place on burgers; top with bacon. Serve on lettuce, if desired.

NUTRIENTS PER SERVING (SERVING SIZE: 1 BURGER WITHOUT EGG)
CALORIES 330   **TOTAL FAT** 23g   **CARBS** 0g   **NET CARBS** 0g   **DIETARY FIBER** 0g   **PROTEIN** 31g

GREEK CHICKEN BURGERS WITH CUCUMBER YOGURT SAUCE

MAKES 4 SERVINGS

½ cup plus 2 tablespoons plain Greek yogurt

½ medium cucumber, peeled, seeded and finely chopped

Juice of ½ lemon

3 cloves garlic, minced, divided

2 teaspoons finely chopped fresh mint *or* ½ teaspoon dried mint

⅛ teaspoon salt

⅛ teaspoon ground white pepper

1 pound ground chicken

3 ounces crumbled feta cheese

4 large kalamata olives, rinsed, patted dry and minced

1 egg

½ teaspoon dried oregano

¼ teaspoon black pepper

Mixed baby lettuce (optional)

1 Combine yogurt, cucumber, lemon juice, 2 cloves garlic, mint, salt and white pepper in medium bowl; mix well. Cover and refrigerate until ready to serve.

2 Combine chicken, feta, olives, egg, oregano, black pepper and remaining 1 clove garlic in large bowl; mix well. Shape mixture into four patties.

3 Spray grill pan with nonstick cooking spray; heat over medium-high heat. Grill patties 5 to 7 minutes per side or until cooked through (165°F).

4 Serve burgers with sauce and mixed greens, if desired.

NUTRIENTS PER SERVING (SERVING SIZE: 1 BURGER AND ¼ OF SAUCE)

CALORIES 260 **TOTAL FAT** 14g **CARBS** 4g **NET CARBS** 3g **DIETARY FIBER** 1g **PROTEIN** 29g

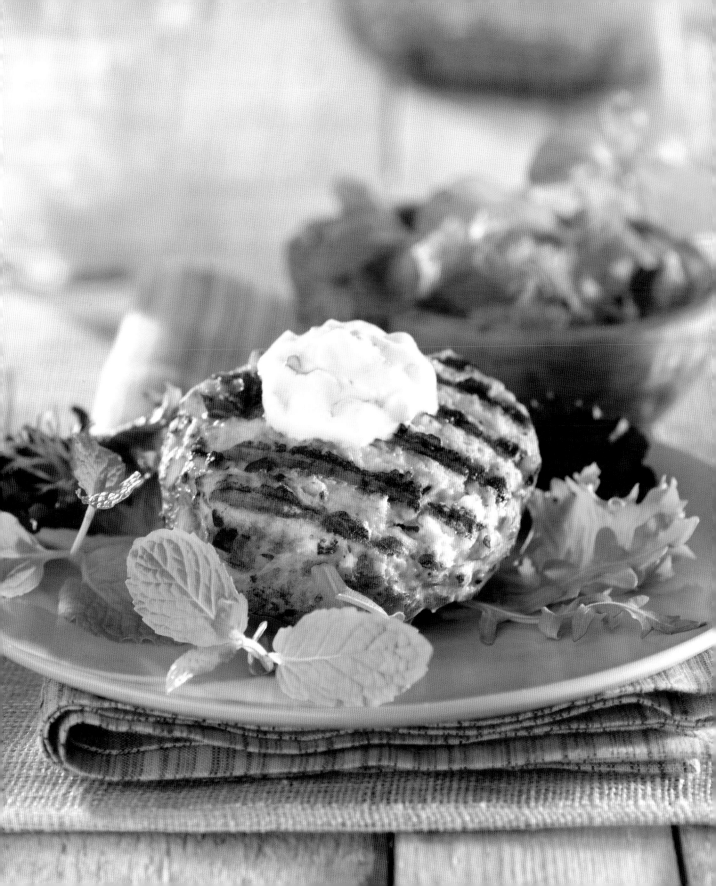

KETO BREAD

MAKES 1 LOAF (16 SLICES)

7 tablespoons butter, divided

2 cups almond flour

3½ teaspoons baking powder

½ teaspoon salt

6 eggs at room temperature, separated*

¼ teaspoon cream of tartar

Discard 1 egg yolk.

1 Preheat oven to 375°F. Generously grease 8×4-inch loaf pan with 1 tablespoon butter. Melt remaining 6 tablespoons butter; cool slightly.

2 Combine almond flour, baking powder and salt in medium bowl. Add melted butter and 5 egg yolks; stir until blended.

3 Place egg whites and cream of tartar in bowl of electric stand mixer; attach whip attachment to mixer. Whip egg whites on high speed 1 to 2 minutes or until stiff peaks form.

4 Stir one third of egg whites into almond flour mixture until well blended. Gently fold in remaining egg whites until thoroughly blended. Scrape batter into prepared pan; smooth top.

5 Bake 25 to 30 minutes or until top is light brown and dry and toothpick inserted into center comes out clean. Cool in pan on wire rack 10 minutes. Remove from pan; cool completely.

NUTRIENTS PER SERVING (SERVING SIZE: 1 SLICE)

CALORIES 156   **TOTAL FAT** 13g   **CARBS** 4g   **NET CARBS** 2g   **DIETARY FIBER** 2g   **PROTEIN** 5g

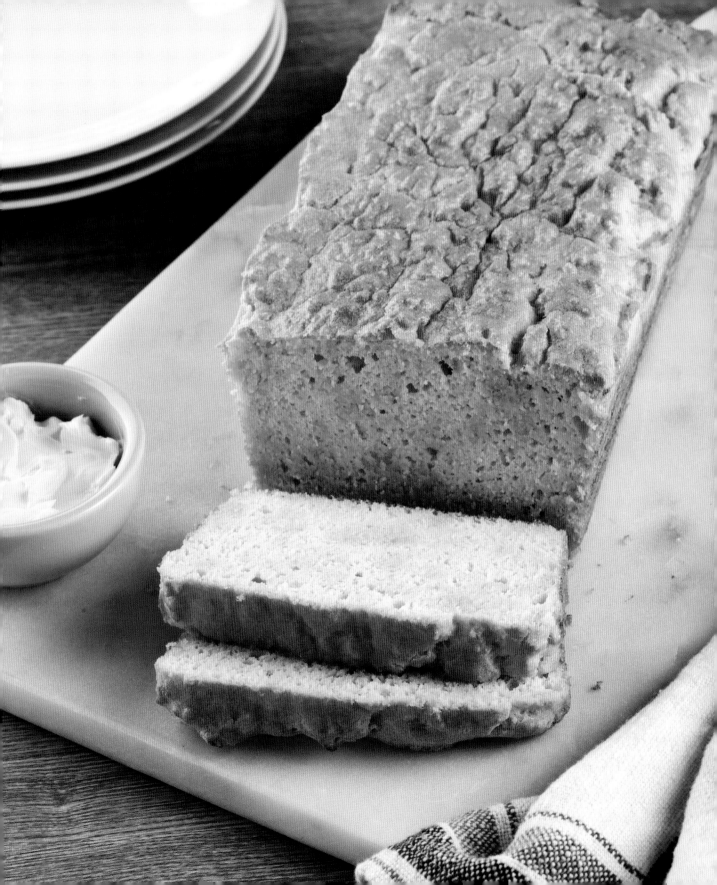

KETO TUNA MELT

MAKES 4 SERVINGS

¾ cup mayonnaise

2 teaspoons lemon juice

1 teaspoon salt

⅛ teaspoon black pepper

1 can (12 ounces) solid white albacore tuna, drained

1 can (12 ounces) chunk light tuna, drained

1 stalk celery, finely chopped (about ½ cup)

¼ cup minced red onion

½ loaf Keto Bread (page 180), cut into 8 slices

8 slices Cheddar cheese

2 tablespoons butter

Optional toppings: tomato slices, avocado slices, red onion rings, pickles and/or lettuce leaves

1 Combine mayonnaise, lemon juice, salt and pepper in large bowl. Add tuna, celery and onion; mix well.

2 Divide tuna among bread slices; top each with cheese. Heat 1 tablespoon butter in large skillet over medium heat until melted. Add half of sandwiches; cover and cook until bread is toasted and cheese is melted. Repeat with remaining butter and sandwiches. Garnish with desired toppings.

NUTRIENTS PER SERVING (SERVING SIZE: 2 SANDWICHES)

CALORIES 980   **TOTAL FAT** 80g   **CARBS** 9g   **NET CARBS** 6g   **DIETARY FIBER** 3g   **PROTEIN** 62g

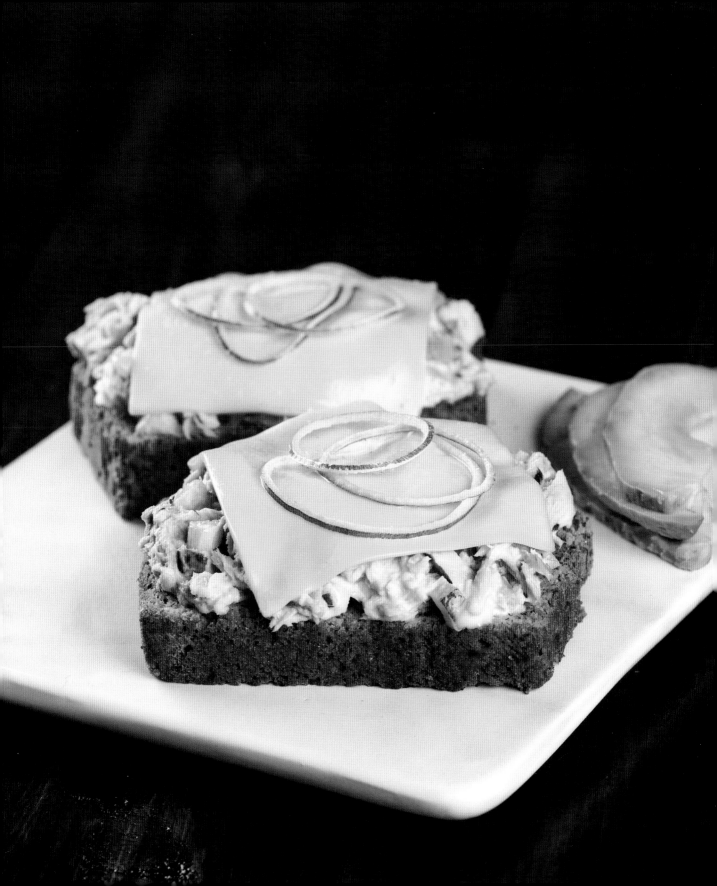

BACON-TOMATO GRILLED CHEESE

MAKES 4 SERVINGS

- 8 slices bacon, cut in half
- 4 slices sharp Cheddar cheese
- 4 slices Gouda cheese
- 4 tomato slices, cut in half
- ½ loaf Keto Bread (page 180), cut into 8 slices
- 1 tablespoon butter

1. Cook bacon in large skillet over medium-high heat until crisp. Remove from skillet; drain on paper towels. Drain fat from skillet; wipe out skillet with paper towels.

2. Layer 1 slice of Cheddar, 1 slice of Gouda, 2 tomato halves and 4 bacon slices between two bread slices. Melt 1 tablespoon butter in same skillet over medium heat. Add sandwiches; cook 3 to 4 minutes or until bottoms are toasted. Flip sandwiches. Reduce heat to medium-low; cover and cook 3 to 4 minutes or until bottoms are toasted and cheese is melted.

NUTRIENTS PER SERVING (SERVING SIZE: 1 SANDWICH)

CALORIES 530 **TOTAL FAT** 45g **CARBS** 10g **NET CARBS** 7g **DIETARY FIBER** 3g **PROTEIN** 27g

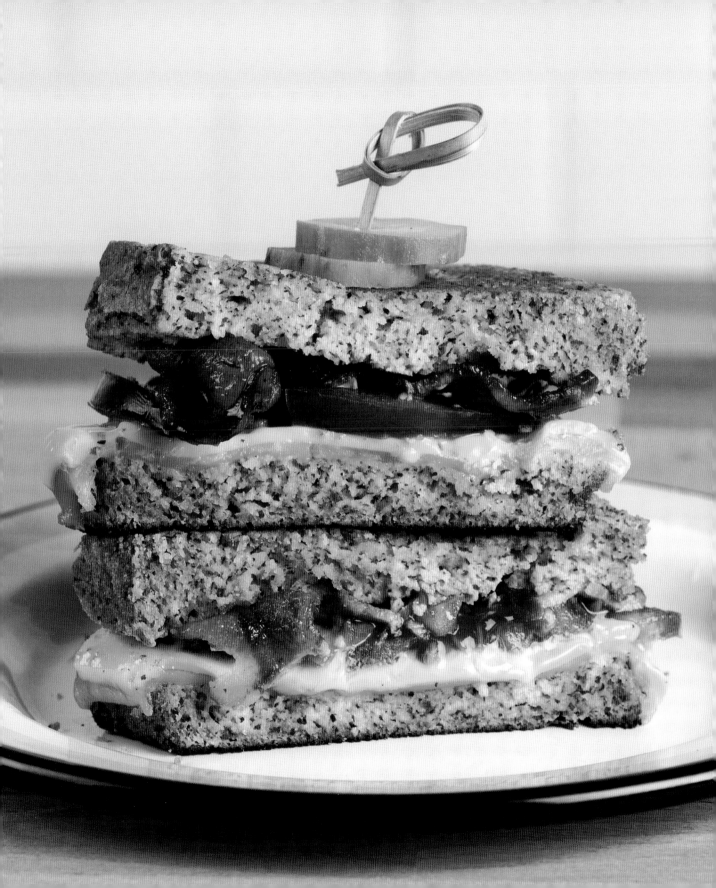

SALMON BURGERS WITH TARRAGON AÏOLI SAUCE

MAKES 4 SERVINGS

TARRAGON AÏOLI SAUCE

- ⅓ cup sour cream
- 1½ tablespoons mayonnaise
- 1 tablespoon milk
- ½ teaspoon dried tarragon
- ¼ teaspoon salt
- ⅛ teaspoon black pepper

BURGER

- 1 can (6 ounces) pink salmon, drained
- ¼ cup almond flour
- ⅓ cup chopped green onions
- ¼ cup chopped fresh cilantro
- 2 egg whites
- 2 tablespoons lime juice
- ¼ teaspoon salt
- ⅛ teaspoon ground red pepper

1 For sauce, combine sour cream, mayonnaise, milk, tarragon, ¼ teaspoon salt and black pepper in medium bowl; stir to blend. Refrigerate until ready to use.

2 For burgers, combine salmon, almond flour, green onions, cilantro, egg whites, lime juice and red pepper in large bowl; mix well.

3 Spray large nonstick skillet with nonstick cooking spray; heat over medium heat. Spoon salmon mixture into four mounds in skillet. Using flat spatula, flatten mounds into patties. Cook 3 minutes per side or until golden. Serve with sauce.

NUTRIENTS PER SERVING (SERVING SIZE: 1 BURGER AND 2 TABLESPOONS SAUCE)

CALORIES 190   **TOTAL FAT** 14g   **CARBS** 6g   **NET CARBS** 4g   **DIETARY FIBER** 2g   **PROTEIN** 11g

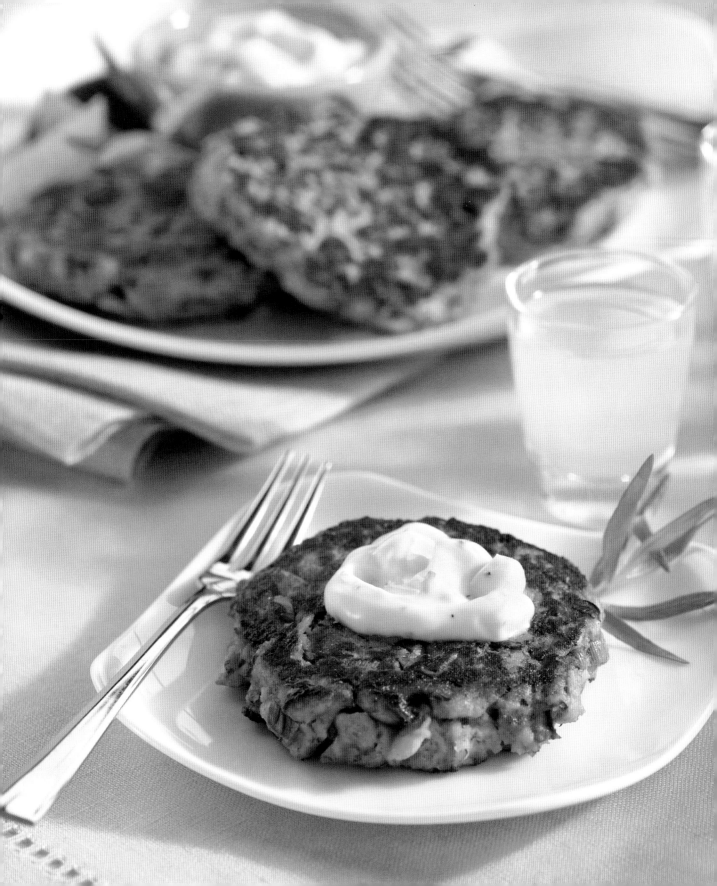

METRIC CONVERSION CHART

VOLUME MEASUREMENTS (dry)

1/8 teaspoon = 0.5 mL
1/4 teaspoon = 1 mL
1/2 teaspoon = 2 mL
3/4 teaspoon = 4 mL
1 teaspoon = 5 mL
1 tablespoon = 15 mL
2 tablespoons = 30 mL
1/4 cup = 60 mL
1/3 cup = 75 mL
1/2 cup = 125 mL
2/3 cup = 150 mL
3/4 cup = 175 mL
1 cup = 250 mL
2 cups = 1 pint = 500 mL
3 cups = 750 mL
4 cups = 1 quart = 1 L

VOLUME MEASUREMENTS (fluid)

1 fluid ounce (2 tablespoons) = 30 mL
4 fluid ounces (1/2 cup) = 125 mL
8 fluid ounces (1 cup) = 250 mL
12 fluid ounces (1 1/2 cups) = 375 mL
16 fluid ounces (2 cups) = 500 mL

WEIGHTS (mass)

1/2 ounce = 15 g
1 ounce = 30 g
3 ounces = 90 g
4 ounces = 120 g
8 ounces = 225 g
10 ounces = 285 g
12 ounces = 360 g
16 ounces = 1 pound = 450 g

DIMENSIONS

1/16 inch = 2 mm
1/8 inch = 3 mm
1/4 inch = 6 mm
1/2 inch = 1.5 cm
3/4 inch = 2 cm
1 inch = 2.5 cm

OVEN TEMPERATURES

250°F = 120°C
275°F = 140°C
300°F = 150°C
325°F = 160°C
350°F = 180°C
375°F = 190°C
400°F = 200°C
425°F = 220°C
450°F = 230°C

BAKING PAN SIZES

Utensil	Size in Inches/Quarts	Metric Volume	Size in Centimeters
Baking or Cake Pan (square or rectangular)	8 × 8 × 2	2 L	20 × 20 × 5
	9 × 9 × 2	2.5 L	23 × 23 × 5
	12 × 8 × 2	3 L	30 × 20 × 5
	13 × 9 × 2	3.5 L	33 × 23 × 5
Loaf Pan	8 × 4 × 3	1.5 L	20 × 10 × 7
	9 × 5 × 3	2 L	23 × 13 × 7
Round Layer Cake Pan	8 × 1½	1.2 L	20 × 4
	9 × 1½	1.5 L	23 × 4
Pie Plate	8 × 1¼	750 mL	20 × 3
	9 × 1¼	1 L	23 × 3
Baking Dish or Casserole	1 quart	1 L	—
	1½ quart	1.5 L	—
	2 quart	2 L	—